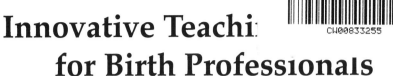

Innovative Teaching
for Birth Professionals

Second Edition

Connie L. Livingston

Praeclarus Press, LLC

www.PraeclarusPress.com

Praeclarus Press, LLC

2504 Sweetgum Lane

Amarillo, Texas 79124 USA

806-367-9950

www.PraeclarusPress.com

DISCLAIMER

The information contained in this publication is advisory only and is not intended to replace sound clinical judgments or individualized patient care. The author disclaims all warranties, whether expressed or implied, including any warranty as the quality, accuracy, safety, or suitability of this information for any particular purpose.

ISBN: 9781939807427

Cover Design: Ken Tackett

Acquisition & Development: Kathleen Kendall-Tackett

Copy Editing: Chris Tackett

Layout & Design: Todd Rollison

Operations: Scott Sherwood

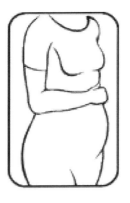

Foreword

All throughout the her-story of childbirth, until the last 80 to 100 years, women attended births of their loved ones, friends, and family, and learned the art of comfort, and about the process of childbirth, as they learned about life, through stories and experience. When we broke this circle of support in childbirth, and moved birth into a medical environment, doctors took over as the decision makers, machines became more valued than tender loving care, and we lost a body of knowledge about how to have a gentle birth with loving support. We also lost the power that birth holds in our lives as a rite of passage from maidenhood to motherhood, and from men to fathers.

Birth became viewed as only a physical process, without valuing and acknowledging the emotional, and for many, the spiritual process of labor, birth, and becoming a parent. The importance was placed on surviving childbirth. It was just a day, so it did not matter if our babies were cut out, sucked out, or pulled out. The value was on having a healthy baby. Women were told to lie down and give their body over to medicine. Your doctor will deliver your baby for you. We have since learned the importance of not only surviving, but thriving in childbirth. Too many women suffer for days and years after having a birth experience, and thus memory, that is distressing, or in too many cases, traumatic. To ensure a positive birth memory, women need continuous support, to have information about all their options, to be an active participant involved in informed decision making, and to be respected and honored at one of life's most amazing and sacred moments.

Providing information, and preparing women and men to understand the process of childbirth, all their options, and how to speak up to give and receive respect is the essential role of quality childbirth education. We no longer live in a time where we will attend many births before our own, and learn about childbirth as a life skill within our families or communities. Birth has become shrouded in fear, and knowledge is lost. So today, good childbirth classes help mothers understand the power and possibilities that birth holds in our lives. Too few people are preparing for childbirth today, and I believe some of that is due to educators failing to teach in a way that inspires, builds confidence in women's bodies, facilitates the release of fears, builds a community, and help women and men to reclaim their power in birth.

How can you pass along this knowledge in your childbirth classes to provide the foundation for a healthy pregnancy, birth, breastfeeding, and postpartum? How can you create classes that are interactive, fun, and allow women and men to awaken their own inner wisdom, and birth the way that honors their beliefs, values, and desires, and builds upon the traditions of the past?

I remember meeting Connie Livingston as a new doula and educator, and being taken with her knowledge and creative approaches to teaching. Her ideas create the space for invigorating and thoughtful discussion honoring each persons' perspective and path to giving birth with love, respect, and dignity. From icebreaker games and toolkits to learning styles, *Innovative Teaching Strategies for Birth* will inspire you with innovative ideas to teach Anatomy and Physiology, the Labor Process, Reviews and Rehearsals, Medications and Interventions, Options and Decision making, Breastfeeding; all that is essential for women and their partners to consider to create a safe, satisfying birth.

Connie's exercises and ideas provide the template to make your childbirth classes not only educational, but exceptional! Even as an educator for 30 years, *Innovative Teaching Strategies for Birth* has rekindled my passion to bring more fun into preparation, teaching, and learning.

Thank you, Connie, for helping us reclaim the wisdom of birth with a toolkit that makes childbirth education the interactive, thought-provoking, life-changing experience it was meant to be to prepare women and men to reclaim childbirth with knowledge. Knowledge is Power!

—Debra Pascali Bonaro

Producer, Orgasmic Birth

Contents

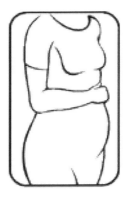

About This Book

It is paradoxical that many educators and parents still differentiate between a time for learning, and a time for play, without seeing the vital connection between them.

—Leo F. Buscaglia, 1924-1998

In our lives, learning takes place in a variety of locations and through a variety of media. There are as many ways to present information as there are learners to absorb it. The key, therefore, is to present information in a way learners will be eager to use and want to learn more. Learning has to be fun and familiar to engage the learner. Passive education disengages the learner.

This book is designed to inspire you to expand teaching practices, become more creative, and ultimately increase your passion for the work you do. By interweaving new and innovative teaching strategies into your childbirth curriculum, you become more excited about teaching and, therefore, pass that excitement on to your class members. You will renew your energy and passion for this work, and that will be reflected to your class.

An anonymous quote I came upon states, "Those who dare to teach, must never cease to learn." My hope is that you are inspired by the tremendous creativity and talent of our fellow birth educators and, no matter how long you have been teaching, you continue to look to each other for motivation. Never stop learning.

—Connie Livingston

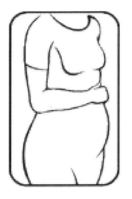

Chapter 1
Teaching Gen X, Y, and Beyond: Group Dynamics

The mediocre teacher tells. The good teacher explains. The superior teacher demonstrates. The great teacher inspires.

—William A. Ward

Creating an environment where learning takes place begins with assessing the needs of the learners. Every family experience with pregnancy, birth, and parenting is unique. Each member brings experiences, relationships, and realities as they are perceived by them to the birth. You, as a birth educator, play a vital role in the family's psychosocial adaptation. This relationship is built on trust, security, validation, caring, and support. Your knowledge about the physiologic and psychosocial processes of pregnancy and parenting, along with a strong referral network, allows for identification of difficulties, misconceptions, misperceptions, or miscommunication during the childbearing years.

The general public's cumulative knowledge has increased in the last 10 years and will continue to double every five years, according to experts. This is partially due to the increased use of the Internet for research. Clients present themselves in childbirth classes and to doulas with a much broader knowledge base. There is an increasing need for more detail in the information they receive, a need for more autonomy in the pregnancy and birthing process, and a need for more information on infant care and parenting styles. Thus, you must not only meet the basic needs described here, but also a higher level of needs.

Maslow's Hierarchy of Needs

Discussions about psychosocial adaptation begin with knowledge of the classic basic survival needs and growth needs characterized by Maslow's Hierarchy of Needs (Maslow, 1943). Simply put, these needs include physiological: air, water, food, shelter, sex, and sleep;

safety: protection from the elements, disease, fear; belongingness and love: feeling cared for and loved; esteem: self-esteem and esteem by others; and self-actualization: realizing potential, "becoming everything you can be," having "peak" experiences of being. (See Diagram 1.1) A closer look at Maslow's Hierarchy reveals these considerations when caring for the expectant parent.

Physiological Needs

Physiological needs are biological needs consisting of needs for oxygen, food, water, and a relatively constant body temperature. They are the strongest of needs because if all needs are deprived, the physiological ones would come first in the person's search for satisfaction.

Diagram 1.1

These needs may become compromised during pregnancy due to morning sickness, gestational diabetes, or during labor itself. The health educator can offer alternatives or suggestions in addition to what the primary caregiver has already suggested. This might include nutritional education, smoking cessation referrals, and adequate hydration.

When teaching in a classroom setting, be aware of the various physiological needs of your class attendees. By providing or having access to water or other drinks, nutritional snacks, adequate restroom facilities, comfortable seating, appropriate room temperature, and scheduled break times, you can optimize the learning potential of your class members.

Safety Needs

When all physiological needs are satisfied and are no longer influencing thoughts and behaviors, the need for security can become active. Some adults have little awareness of their security needs except in times of emergency or periods of disorganization in the social structure. Adults may feel vulnerable during the childbearing experience, especially if they have not attended childbirth education classes or have never been in the hospital setting. We witness in children the signs of insecurity and the need to be safe. Nurturing plays a key role with this need. Likewise, expectant parents seem to respond to this nurturing and feeling of safety. Birth educators are, by their very nature, nurturers. Clients may have an increased satisfaction with their birth after, for example, taking childbirth education classes, or having a midwife or doula-supported birth.

Safety needs are vital in preparing a classroom for learning. Safety issues in childbirth classes include adequate emergency exits, lighting, and security in parking lots or parking garages near the facility, access to a phone or cell service to check on the other children of class members, cleanliness of the facility, easy access to the room, and handicap accessibility.

Needs of Love, Affection, and Belonging

When the needs for safety and for physiological well-being are satisfied, the next area of needs for love, affection, and belonging can emerge. Maslow states that people seek to overcome feelings of loneliness and alienation (Maslow, 1943). This involves both giving and receiving love, affection, and the sense of belonging. The expectant mother and the father or partner have strong needs for love and affection during this tumultuous time. Birth educators can assist the father or partner in meeting the emotional needs of the mother, while also assisting with the ever-challenging physical needs.

Likewise, in childbirth classes, in order for each class member to feel free enough to open up to the group and facilitate group cohesion, they should be made to feel welcome. From the time they walk into the room, they should feel like they belong. A simple handshake and a "Welcome" will set the stage for accepting their place in the group. Throughout the learning experience, take time to connect with each member, always making them feel like they are special and are a vital part of a classroom.

Needs for Esteem

When the first three needs are satisfied, the needs for esteem may become dominant. This involves both self-esteem and the feedback a person receives from others. Humans have a need for a stable, firmly based, high level of self-respect, and respect from others. When these needs are satisfied, the person may feel self-confident and valuable as a person in the world. When these needs are not satisfied, the person may feel inferior, weak, helpless, and worthless. Nothing is more important in the entire scope of childbearing than respect and trust, not only from the members of a childbirth class series, but also from the care provider. The relationship, especially in maternity care, affects the mother and, subsequently, her entire family for many years. It can influence how confident the mother and father are in caring for their children, thus effecting another generation.

Judgement, by words, body language or facial expressions, is never an appropriate response by an educator to a comment or opinion from a client or class member. Regardless of their comments, each member of the class is important and must be treated as such. Remember, an educator's role is to empower the class, not control it. By controlling, the educator removes the power from the class. This could leave them with a lower self-esteem which, in turn, could lead to feelings of not being able to make decisions for themselves, let alone their children.

Needs for Self-Actualization

When all previous needs are satisfied, then and only then, are the needs for self-actualization activated. Maslow describes self-actualization as a person's need to be and do that for which the person was born. A musician must make music, an artist needs to paint, a poet must write–and mothers need to nurture their babies. The person needing self-actualization feels on-edge, tense, lacking something: in short, restless. If a person is hungry, unsafe, not loved or accepted, or lacking self-esteem, it is very easy to see why the person is restless. It is not always clear what a person wants when there is a need for self-actualization. Communication is once again a key component.

Pregnancy and birth are important events in every culture. Yet, attitudes toward these processes vary considerably, even within one society. Competing views of pregnancy exist in American culture: one views pregnancy as a "crisis," and the other regards it as a normal rite of passage. Each of these attitudes have differing protocols and when allowed to go to completion, impacts a woman's life differently. Rather than rely on an attitude steeped in tradition, it may be best to prescribe to a birth protocol substantiated in research-based fact. Care should be taken to respect the culture and diversity of the family, as well as the informed choices a mother makes based on her basic needs. By helping expectant parents become aware of their resources, and supporting them in their decision making, maternal health providers can minimize a great deal of the stress associated with this rite of passage.

How People Retain Information

According to Dale's Cone of Experience, we retain information from a variety of mediums (Dale, 1969) (See Diagram 1.2). While the validity of this pyramid has been questioned, it is still true that when choosing teaching strategies, the birth educator should keep in mind the different learning styles. For maximum knowledge retention, be certain to combine various teaching strategies that touch on all of the active learning skills.

Being an effective educator involves understanding how adults learn best. Adults have unique needs as learners. The field of adult learning was pioneered by Malcom Knowles (Knowles, 1998). He identified the following characteristics of adult learners:

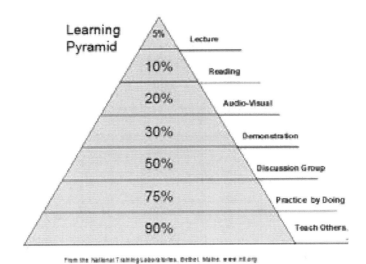

Diagram 1.2

- **Adults are autonomous and self-direct-ed.** They need to be free to direct themselves. Educators must actively involve adult partici-pants in the learning process and serve as facili-tators for them. Specifically, educators must get participants' perspectives about what topics to cover and let them work on projects reflecting their interests. They should allow the partici-pants to assume responsibility for presentations and group leadership. Thus, group work and "show-and-tell" sessions work well with adults.

- **Adults are relevancy-oriented and accumulate a vast storehouse of life experiences and knowledge that may include work-related activities, family experiences, and previous education.** Connecting the life skills learned in childbirth education classes with their personal knowledge and experience base enhances both their knowledge and retention.

- **Adults are goal-oriented.** During the first night of class, adults appreciate an overview of what is to be learned, plus organization and clearly defined goals

- **Adults are practical, focusing on the aspects of a lesson most useful to them in life.** Educators should examine ways the tools and techniques learned in class will be useful to them in the future.

- **As do all learners, adults need to be shown respect.** Educators must acknowledge the wealth of experiences adult participants bring to the classroom. Adults should be treated as equals and allowed to voice their opinions freely in class. They should not be talked down to or have class content read to them from notes.

Motivation of Adult Learners

Another aspect of adult learning is *motivation*. There are many influences on educational motivation, including:

- **Social Relationships.** People learning or going to a class want to make new friends and interact with like-minded individuals.

- **External Expectations.** Expectant parents want to know what will be happening in the birthplace and how to work with their caregivers (nurse, midwife, or physician) to meet mutual goals.

- **Personal Advancement.** Expectant parents often have goals, such as how to achieve a certain portion of the birth plan, with flexibility built into the plan.

- **Cognitive Interest.** Pregnancy and childbirth books and websites are helpful, but to satisfy an inquiring mind about the mechanism of birth and the method for working with the contraction, classes become the primary learning mechanism for many parents.

Barriers and Motivation

Adults have many responsibilities that they must balance against the demands of learning, and often these responsibilities are seen as barriers against participating in learning. Some of these barriers include lack of time, money, confidence, or interest; lack of information about opportunities to learn; scheduling problems; low literacy; "red tape"; and problems with childcare and transportation.

The best way to motivate adult learners is simply to enhance their reasons for enrolling in the childbirth education class and decrease the barriers. Learn why your students are enrolled (the motivators), and discover what is keeping them from learning (the barriers). With this information, you are better equipped to plan motivating strategies and infuse them into your teaching.

Teaching Tips for Effective Educators

As educators, we must remember that learning occurs within each individual as a continual process throughout life. People learn at different speeds, so it is natural for them to be anxious or nervous when faced with a new learning situation. Positive reinforcement can enhance learning, as can proper timing of the instruction. Praise, encouragement, and other methods of positive reinforcement are the keys to the self-actualization of our expectant participants.

There are three critical elements of learning that must be addressed to ensure participants learn. These elements are motivation, reinforcement, and retention

Motivation

If the participant does not recognize the need for the information, all of your efforts to assist the participant to learn will be lost. You must establish rapport with participants and prepare them for learning. This provides motivation.

In addition, participants need specific knowledge of their learning results (feedback). Demonstrations with return demonstrations or practice labor rehearsals are effective methods to provide feedback.

Reinforcement

Reinforcement is a necessary part of the teaching and learning process; through it, you encourage correct modes of behavior and performance.

- *Positive reinforcement* is normally used by educators who are teaching participants new skills.

As the name implies, positive reinforcement is "good" and reinforces "good" (or positive) behavior.

- *Negative reinforcement* may be used by some educators teaching a new skill or new information. However, with childbirth education, suggestions for performing a skill are preferred over negative reinforcement.

Retention

Expectant parents should retain information learned in childbirth classes and be able to apply this information during the labor process. To help them retain what is taught, they need to see a purpose for the information. This purpose can be demonstrated to them in the form of videos of labor, or by using guest speakers who have recently gone through the birth experience. Retention by the participants is directly affected by their amount of practice during the learning. Approximately one-third of the childbirth education class should be set aside for the practice of new techniques or review of previously learned techniques.

Examining Views and Biases

In maternity care, there seems to be the medical model and the holistic model, with an area in-between.

24

The medical model sees birth as a potential crisis needing to be managed for safety. The holistic model of birth acknowledges the language of women's bodies, and sees the weaving of body, mind, and spirit as an essential element for empowerment.

Women have trusted their bodies in the birthing process since the beginning of mankind. They have embraced birth as a passage from womanhood to motherhood. These women see birth as a dramatic life-altering event. Many childbirth activists and educators believe that with the industrial era, women were convinced machines and technology were more adept at guiding them through labor than their own instincts. After all, it was technology that enhanced transportation, created financial stability, and won wars. It was a natural assumption that technology would bring healthier babies.

Educators often fall between the holistic and medical model. They teach "preparedness" for childbirth, which is objectively teaching about labor and birth. Ideally, biases should be kept in check. Biases may be in the form of body language, or even voice inflection, if the information is given orally. When considering a cesarean section for failure to progress, for example, the caregiver's words, "You've been at 8 cm for a long time" can be said many different ways. Some body cues and voice inflections would be very persuasive toward a cesarean, while others would be very matter-of-fact and be interpreted as simply giving information.

Dimensions of Learning and Learner Preferences

We have examined the various basic needs of adult learners and the importance of retaining the information. Another important aspect to consider is how adult learners prefer to learn. In other words, each adult learner responds in a different way to each teaching strategy used.

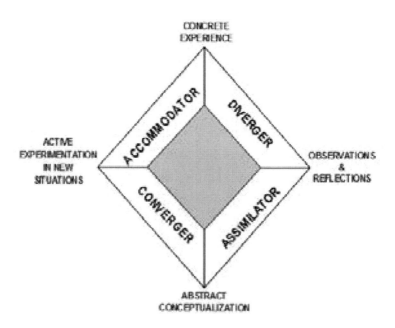

Diagram 1.3. Adapted from Fry. R. & Kolb. D. [1976]. *Experiential learning theory and learning experiences in liberal arts.* California Management Review, p.18.

26

According to Kolb, there are four dimensions to the learning process and four basic preferences for learning (Kolb, 1984, 1985). Dimensions of Learning refer to the pathway through the learning process. As learners journey through each step on the path, they will have certain preferences for the type of strategy used in the four dimensions of learning (See Diagram 1.3). Learners typically can tolerate learning styles which differ from what they prefer as long as their styles are also addressed.

When preparing your curriculum, you should examine teaching strategies along with the content of the curriculum to meet the needs of all of your learners. With properly chosen strategies, you can ensure the greatest retention level from the participants.

In order to explain the dimensions of learning, we will take a sample subject, pelvic rocking, and walk through the various dimensions.

- **Concrete Experience** — When the instructor demonstrates the pelvic rocking technique as a stretching exercise to the class and the class, in turn, returns the demonstration.

- **Observations and Reflections**—Each learner then interprets the experience doing the pelvic rocking exercise.

- **Abstract Conceptualization**—The learner may conclude that with adequate practice of pelvic rocking, the lower back will be more relaxed and more capable of supporting the added strain on her lower back towards the end of pregnancy.

- **Active Experimentation in New Situations**—The learner remembers the pelvic rocking technique and considers it during back labor. She concludes that pelvic rocking will pull the baby off her lower back and gravity can help to turn the posterior baby. She will use pelvic rocking for this new situation.

Understanding Learner Preferences

Once the pathway of learning is understood, then you must address the individual's preferences for learning. Each individual learner usually prefers teaching strategies reflecting one or two of the dimensions of learning. Below are the types of learner preferences and appropriate teaching strategies for each.

- **Accommodators**—Like to experience situations and prefer feedback, are planners and doers, adapt well to situa-tions, and may be known as risk-takers. Suggested teaching strategies: role-play, return demonstration, audio-visual materials.

- **Divergers**—Prefer less detail-oriented curriculum; are very imaginative; do not focus on details, but focus on the end product; need time to process the information given; and explore feelings by watching and listening. Suggested teaching strategies: reading, discussion, brainstorming, and small group work.

- **Assimilators**—Choose to draw their own inferences, create their own theories without regard to practicality, prefer information given in an organized manner, and learn from watching others. Suggested teaching strategies: reading, lecture, charts, graphs, models, and working alone.

- **Convergers**—Need structure and order, are task-oriented and not emotional, prefer a linear view of material, and prefer technical tasks. Suggested teaching strategies include practical reading, group reports, and discussion (Brady, 2013).

Since it is likely your childbirth education class will be made up of several individuals, each with their own learning styles and preferences, it becomes imperative to address each class members' needs throughout the childbirth class series. This will improve your effectiveness, as well as the impact of the birthing class on each participant.

The Group Process

Teaching individuals and teaching a group have both similarities and differences. Teaching individuals, in the case of private childbirth classes with one or two couples, typically implies these individuals have sought out the educator for a particular reason, and feel a small group is a beneficial learning environment for them. In addition to having fundamental knowledge of the material, teaching a group of 8 to 12 couples requires the organizational and juggling skills of a business person.

In a group, there are many different personalities (Nichols & Humenick, 2000). Some personalities will make teaching and learning fun and enjoyable. Other personalities will be barriers to learning and will create a challenge for teaching. Occasionally, some of the challenging personalities will be strong and forceful. These individuals typically need attention. Remember, you are the facilitator for all of the learners.

Types of People in a Group

- **Info Seeker.** May monopolize the conversation by asking a lot of questions.

- **Opinion Seeker.** May want to play one person's opinion (often a physician) against the educator, or may poll the class to help make their own decisions.

- **Info Giver.** Participates well in the class. May feel the need to provide copious amounts of information.

- **Opinion Giver.** May over-participate by being opinionated.

- **Follower**. Is often quiet. Goes along with the crowd or may use you as role model.

- **Aggressor**. Has different opinions about how class should be run, the content in the class, or about how labor/birth should proceed. Often vocal and difficult to cope with.

- **Blocker.** May also be the aggressor. May change subject and encourage going off on tangents.

- **Playboy**. May make off-color jokes about partner or subject matter, or laugh at the concepts. Loves attention.

- **Dominator**. The "co-educator." Enjoys sharing experiences of previous birth experiences, or information learned from books or television.

- **ZZZ**. So bored with the class that they fall asleep, or so tired from the days' stressors, they feel totally relaxed.

Choosing Teaching Strategies

The best way to choose the teaching strategies for various topics in a childbirth class is to evaluate the learning through completed class evaluations after all the classes have been taught. This method is ideal for the educator already involved in teaching classes. However, for the inexperienced educator, this is not the ideal.

Choosing a teaching strategy can be a difficult choice, given all of the different types of strategies (See Diagram 1.4). Strategies should be used to invigorate the learner, stimulate learning, and make the experience enjoyable.

Lecture, models, charts, and handouts are preferred strategies for presenting information to learners for the first time. Using a combination of these four strategies enables you to verbally introduce and explain the material. These strategies make the information more concrete and real by using models, charts, slides, and photographs for further explanation. By providing handouts or other written materials to take with them, all the learners needs are addressed and, thus, the way is paved to achieving optimum learning potential of class members.

The learner who likes structure, and tends to be more analytical in nature, seems to like teaching strategies, such as diagrams, charts, graphs, as well as lecture.

Demonstrations, alone or accompanied by return demonstrations, can further illustrate a point made in the class and enhance the learner retention of the skill. Likewise, the use of videos, audio recordings, and some television shows found on public broadcasting stations and cable may validate information previously given and reinforce a concept. It is wise to preview any television program for content and record the show for use in the classroom (with permission, if necessary). In this way, you can be sure that the information you wish to present is accurate and appropriate.

Homework assignments, including worksheets, reporting on website content, or book reading, may also be used to expand on what was learned in class. It can also be used to show the learner where education resources are for future references. Labor rehearsals are a great tool to quiz the class on what they have learned, and assess the areas that need further instruction from you.

Buzz groups, brainstorming, questionnaires, call and response, and Q/A (Question and Answer) sessions can assist you in evaluating a learner's knowledgebase on a particular topic. These can be invaluable in setting the parameters of how deep to go into a subject in the time allotted. Icebreakers may also be used to evaluate the learner, but on a slightly lighter level. Values clarification is an exercise that encourages the class members to examine their views on various subjects. An example would be if you ask a series of questions in which each class member needs to respond with a, "strongly agree," "agree," "unsure," "disagree," or "strongly disagree." These teaching strategies also promote class involvement and group interaction that are essential aspects to class development.

Discussions provide an avenue for sharing knowledge and concerns with the other members of the group. Group-centered discussion is simply allowing the group to facilitate and guide the topics at hand, enabling each to add to the discussion, if they wish. You may also wish to have a select group of individuals lead a panel discussion, such as other birth educators, doulas, midwives, physicians, or a combination. Class members who have previously given birth can also act as a guest panel for those who have not.

Case discussions, problem-solving, experience sharing, and guided discussions all lead to stimulating conversations with adult learners. Debating needs to be used sparingly, and with a great deal of control on your part, so as to not leave the impression that someone lost the debate. This may lower the self-esteem of the one who "lost."

Discussions can become intense, so it is wise to alternate a "heavy" topic or teaching strategy with a "lighter" one. Field trips (tours of Labor and Delivery), role playing, guided imagery and visualization, simulation, journals, drawing or art exercises, cartoons, and illustrations tend to appeal to the more emotional learner. Be cautious when using imagery and visualizations with your clients, however, because some cultures and religions fobid that type of activity. Certainly, no educator wishes to offend any class members.

Types of Teaching Strategies

Brainstorming	Questionnaire
Buzz Groups	Storytelling
Demo/Return Demonstration	Call and Response
Group-Centered Discussion	Role Playing
Panel Discussion	Simulation
Case Discussion	Values Clarification
Labor Rehearsal	Imagery/Visualization
Problem-Solving Discussion	Grab Bag
Experience-Sharing Discussion	Goal Setting
Guided Discussion	Worksheets
Graffiti Sheets	Workbooks
Field Trip	Books
Games	Journals
Interview	Handouts
Lecture	Drawing/Art
Television	Slides
Debate	Videos
Non-Verbal Exercises	Charts
Peer Instruction	Models
Question/Answer	Photographs
Cartoons/Illustrations	Audio Recordings
Diagrams	Graphs

Diagram 1.4. Nichols, F. & Humenick, S. (2000). *Childbirth education: practice, research, and theory. 2nd.* Ed. Philadelphia: W.B. Saunders.

Games, interviews, storytelling, and non-verbal exercises are other teaching strategies that tend to be more fun and non-threatening, while promoting group interaction.

Exhibits, grab-bags, and field trips appeal to the learner who prefers to see and touch items in order to help retain information. For this learner, words are not enough. Pictures are adequate.

However, for the greatest learning potential, they prefer to see and feel the actual items or equipment (Brady, 2013).

Evaluating Videos: DVD and YouTube

For the visual learner, and for a change of teaching strategy, videos can be a useful tool for the birth educator. DVDs from companies, such as Injoy Video, can supplement the curriculum content that educators develop, and help doulas reinforce concepts presented at prenatal visits.

Using videos has increased exponentially over the years with the ease and availability of DVDs, and also free videos from YouTube. These videos can reinforce and supplement reading and lecture material, provide greater comprehension for the diverse learning styles and also promote perception of educator competence.

DVDs that are purchased and professional are also expensive, so ask these 10 questions when evaluating DVDs for purchase for educational use:

1. Was the message of the video evidence-based?

2. Did the message of the video demonstrate informed consent?

3. Could the video be used for teens?

4. Was the length of the video appropriate for use in a class or doula consult?

5. Was the message of the video biased?

6. Is the cost of the video outside of the budget?

7. Would the video be best used in a specialty class or situation?

8. Could the video be used in any type of class or situation?

9. Was the message of the video clear?

10. Would this be a wise purchase and enhance educational effectiveness?

YouTube is an extremely powerful tool, and free. With about 3 billion videos viewed daily, educators of all types use YouTube to introduce students to concepts and add to the curriculum presented.

Birth educators and doulas should preview You-Tube videos prior to recommending them. A preview can eliminate surprises and can help the educator be confident about content, whether it is posted on social media platforms or recommended within the context of a class. For simplification, a birth educator could create a YouTube channel and refer clients to that channel, where previewed content can be stored.

The knowledge that clients bring with them can greatly affect their learning experiences. Exaggerated stories, old wives' tales, as well as the media's perspective on labor and birth should be addressed. This will enable new information to be connected and reorganized with the learner (Stadtlander, 2013).

Many hospitals seek Magnet Status. The Magnet Recognition Program®, developed by the American Nurses Credentialing Center, or ANCC, recognizes health care organizations for excellence in all aspects of nursing service. For the childbirth educator or doula working within the hospital setting, applying a nursing theory to the education demonstrates the childbirth educator/doula's contribution to nursing excellence. One nursing theory that is particularly applicable is the Virginia Henderson theory, often called the "Definition of Nursing" (Waller-Wise, 2013).

Henderson's theory recognizes that some "patients" are not ill, but are experiencing normal life occurrences within the hospital. In fact, Henderson indicates that in her theory through the statement: "nursing care is providing knowledge and confidence for the young mother." Henderson's 14 Basic Human Needs are easily applied to the birthing process.

1. Breathe normally.

2. Eat and drink adequately.

3. Eliminate body wastes.

4. Move and maintain desirable postures.

5. Sleep and rest.

6. Select suitable clothes: dress and undress.

7. Maintain body temperature within a normal range by adjusting clothing and modifying the environment.

8. Keep the body clean and well-groomed, and protect the integument.

9. Avoid dangers in the environment, and avoid injuring others.

10. Communicate with others in expressing emotions, needs, fears, or opinions.

11. Worship according to one's faith.

12. Work in such a way that there is a sense of accomplishment.

13. Play or participate in various forms of recreation.

14. Learn, discover, or satisfy the curiosity that leads to normal developmental and health, and use the available health facilities.

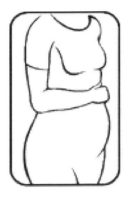

Chapter 2
Introductions and Icebreakers

A good teacher, like a good entertainer, first must hold his audience's attention. Then he can teach his lesson.

—Hendrik John Clarke

The first night of class can be stressful for some expectant parents. Thrust into a group of other parents-to-be may be a great way to begin friendships for some, while inhibiting to others. Icebreakers encourage an air of openness and trust within the classroom setting, and help overcome the initial uncomfortable feeling some people have when first placed in a group (Chlup & Collins, 2010).

There are many useful icebreaker lists currently on the Internet. One of the best was created by Wayne State University in Detroit, Michigan (www.lc.wayne. edu/pdf/icebreakers_teambuilders.pdf). The list includes a wide variety of icebreakers that can be used in teen or adult childbirth education classes.

This chapter contains many tried-and-true icebreakers that have actually been used in childbirth education classes. These icebreakers can be used the first night of class, or you may wish to use a group cohesion activity for the first couple nights of class. As with all the ideas in this handbook, we invite you to be creative and alter these icebreakers to meet your particular needs.

The Toilet Paper Revelation

For this icebreaker, you will need a full roll of toilet tissue. Begin at one point in the group and instruct the members pass it around. Invite each class member to take as many squares as they feel necessary. They must take at least one. (A joke might be made that this particular roll of toilet tissue has nothing to do with the stocking of the restroom used by the class). Once the entire class has their squares of tissue, tell them that for every square they took, they must say something about themselves. Suggestions would be to have them state their name, due zone, caregiver, place of delivery, hobbies, profession, etc.

A nice twist to this icebreaker is to have the expectant mother say something about her partner for every toilet paper square she took. Then, invite the partner to do the same. Often, it is easier for class members to introduce their partners rather than to talk about themselves. What is also nice is to ask the class members to save one square of tissue for stating something about their partner the other class members would not know about just by looking at him or her.

Post-It Notes™

When couples arrive at class, they receive a Post-It Note™ on which to write their one-word response to the phrase "Childbirth Is _____." The participants are asked to fill in the blank and then post their note on the board. They should be encouraged to write down the first thing that comes to mind. The board is divided into two sections: emotional and physical responses to birth. Since responses usually include words like pain, miracle, scary, and joy, you can lead a discussion on the importance of attending not only to the physical needs of the mother, but also the emotional ones.

In most cases, the emotional needs should be addressed first because they could affect the progress of the physical side of labor. This is a great opportunity for you to discuss the *Fear-Tension-Pain Cycle*, and note how labor will slow down or stop when the mother is fearful. Then the physical side of labor, the pain, should be looked at further. A discussion on the benefits of doula care to ease the fear, tension, and ultimately the pain perception can be addressed as well.

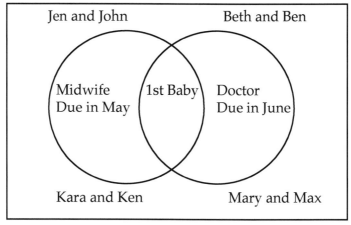

Diagram 2.1

Venn Diagrams

When the couple or individuals arrive to class, they find newsprint papers posted around the room. The number of papers will vary with the number of people or couples in the class. The couples/individuals first names or full names are listed in the four corners. Upon arrival at the class, the couple looks for their names on one of the newsprint sheets; that is their group. Each group chooses someone to write down the information. Under each name, the spokesperson for the group writes down facts on each individual or couple. They list things such as their caregiver, due date, place they will deliver, their job, or anything else they want to share. In the center, they point to things they all have in common (See Diagram 2.1).

On each side, they can list the things that some of the group members have in common. The diagram below gives an example of what to put in the center of the newsprint pages.

This is an excellent icebreaker to use for large groups. It enables the large group to be divided into smaller groups that are much easier to bond. Any exercise such as this allows the group members to begin to share and find commonalities.

What Color Do You Have?

Group activities are essential to create a cohesive environment for learning. The first time you split a class up into groups, a certain level of awkwardness arises. Class members feel reluctant to choose the group in which they will participate. By utilizing this technique, you are able to avoid some of the confusion of where each class member should go.

Purchase solid color ceramic coffee mugs in a variety of colors for about a $1.00 each at a dollar store or other discount stores. When the class participants arrive, tell them to select one mug per couple or individual (if teaching individuals). During the class, use the mug colors to separate people into small groups— either their group has to have all one color for a group sharing, or for the next group sharing, you might tell them that all the mug colors have to be different. The combination of colors is endless. For a small class, you might only use two colors; for a bigger class, you might use three, four, or five colors. Small sharing groups are three to four people, and larger sharing groups are six to eight people.

"What Color Do You Have?" is a fun way to do a group activity. It actually may be cheaper than buying disposable cups for a class, and the participants have an inexpensive "souvenir" from their class. If you are a birth professional trainer and feeling generous and/ or creative, you may wish to put a few things in the mug, like a highlighter marker, mints, or chocolates, affirmations, or a secret homework assignment. You could even put a number on the bottom of the mug for a drawing. If you are teaching a childbirth class, you may wish to substitute the mug with colored water bottles they could use throughout the class, and on into their labor and delivery.

Nametag Swap

In preparing for the arrival of the class members on the first day of class, put the nametags of the class participants on a table. The nametags should be placed in pairs, keeping the couples together. When the couples arrive, instruct them to pick a pair of nametags that is not their own.

When all the nametags have been chosen, tell the class to find the couple who has their nametags. Once they find them, they need to interview that couple to learn more about them. Some questions would be to ask their due date, place of delivery, caregiver, occupation (if appropriate), hobbies, and more. Each will only have to do the interviewing once, interviewing the couple who chose their name. Once the interviews are complete, the couples are asked to introduce the couple to the class whose nametags they've chosen. The nametags then return to their correct owners.

Classmate Scavenger Hunt

On an entire sheet of 8 ½ x 11 paper, make a large table with four columns and five rows. Inside each box of the table, type or write common descriptive characteristics of the participants in a childbirth education class, such as "Goes to Your Doctor," "Has the Same Due Date as You," or "Has Blue Eyes" (See Diagram

2.2). Of course, you can use whatever characteristics you would like. Make enough copies for each participant of the class. Have each participant write the name of the class member next to their corresponding characteristic until all the boxes have a name in them. Use this icebreaker as an effective method for learning more about class participants.

Has the same due date as you.	Has blue eyes.	Mom's partner is blonde.	Is having a girl.
Has other children.	Did not have morning sickness.	Has had a previous cesarean.	The nursery is completely done.
Has experienced Braxton-Hicks contractions.	Craves a certain food.	Will go to the same hospital as you.	Has hired a birth doula.
Has hired a postpartum doula.	Has been on bedrest.	Downloaded the same pregnancy app.	Is having twins or multiples.
Is having a boy.	Is seeing a midwife.	Will be having a home birth.	Has the same doctor as you.

Diagram 2.2

Nametag Personality Drawings

When the class members arrive for the first class, have blank labels or nametag cards on a table and colored markers or pencils available. Each class member should make a nametag

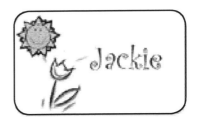

Diagram 2.3

reflecting their personality. The following example would indicate that Jackie is bright and cheerful and loves life (See Diagram 2.3). When the class members have completed their nametags, members then introduce themselves and explain a little about the nametags they created and why the nametag applies to them.

Couples' Interview

If you wish to introduce some class interaction, yet feel large group activities would not be the best option, you may want to suggest a "couples' interview." The couples are presented with a topic for discussion and write down the answers on a piece of paper for reference. One couple asks questions of the other and vice-versa. An example of this activity is to address the subject of induction. Some questions the interviewing couple may ask are:

1. When do you think it is appropriate to induce labor?

2. Under what circumstances would you choose to have labor induced?

3. How do you think labor is started?

4. What concerns, if any, would you have if your caregiver suggests induction?

5. What are some things you have heard about inducing labor naturally?

Depending on the subject and the sensitivity of the issue being discussed, you can choose to have the answers addressed to the entire group. If the questions are of a sensitive nature, you may wish to look at the answers, and then randomly speak to the concerns, or make clarifications on the possible misinformation, without noting publicly from whom the answers came.

You may also wish to write questions on the board, provide handouts with the questions on them, or allow the interviewer to create their own questions on the subject. This activity can be used to discuss a wide variety of topics, and it appeals to those who prefer small-group activities instead of a large group or straight lecture.

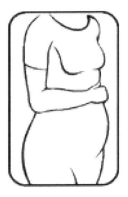

Chapter 3
Anatomy and Physiology

It's not what is poured into a student that counts, but what is planted.

—Linda Conway

Assessing the Learner's Readiness to Learn

In most areas of the United States and Canada, expectant women and their partners have many choices surrounding their birth experiences. This concept of choice, almost always presented as informed choice, began with the childbirth movement in the 1950s. Proponents of women-centered

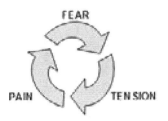

Diagram 3.1

birth advocated a woman's educated choice in birth practices. This ultimately led some physicians, including Grantly Dick-Read and Ferdinand Lamaze, to reintroduce the birth partner or husband, or coach, into the birth environment. Both Dick-Read (Bing, 1994) and Lamaze (Karmel, 2005) suggested a woman in labor builds up tensions because of fear of the unknown. The tensions and fear create an antagonistic effect on the body's muscles causing pain, hence the Fear-Tension-Pain Cycle (See Diagram 3.1). Birth partners play a significant role in breaking this cycle.

Dick-Read proposed education would help women to comprehend the mechanism of labor, allaying their fears, easing tensions, and reducing pain. Lamaze, having observed Russian doctors Nicolaiev and Velvovsky, created the psychoprophylactic method (*psycho* meaning "mind" and *prophylactic* meaning "prevention"). With education as a key component, psychoprophylaxis sought to prevent the mind from dwelling on the intensity of the contractions through a combination of education and techniques, including relaxation, massage or effleurage, focusing, and breathing.

In the 1960s and 1970s, women embraced this more natural way to have their babies (Baldwin, 1995; Bean, 1974; Bing, 1994; Bradley, 2008; Kitzinger, 1979; Kitzinger, 2004). This was in sharp contrast to previous methods of birth in industrialized countries, which included medically induced unconsciousness during labor, and birth with emotional and physical detachment from both this life-changing process and the newborn (Karmel, 2005).

In a discussion about pain, the different types of pain and labor, it is important to point out that pain in labor is:

Purposeful (in that the stretching of the uterine muscles, ligaments, and cervix produce pain);

Anticipated (everyone has heard that there is some pain associated with childbirth);

Intermittent (it is not consistent like a headache or when a bone is broken; it comes and goes with rest periods); and

Normal (unlike other pain, it is normal to have pain during childbirth; it is not a signal that something is wrong; Amis & Green, 2014).

Along with a discussion about pain should be an acknowledgement of possible tocophobia, or the fear of childbirth (Dick-Read, 2013). The fear of childbirth, nearly worldwide, is possibly linked to the perception of no control, and lack of belief in one's own body to give birth physiologically and safely. Tocophobia is characterized by intense fear and anxiety. Primary tocophobia affects nulliparous women to a degree that they may not want to become pregnant. Secondary to-cophobia is associated with a previous traumatic birth experience, catastrophic birth outcome, or even with a physiologic birth with no physical complications. Anxiety and stress lead to secretion of stress hormones, such as epinephrine. Stress hormones cause uterine muscle hypoxia, interruption in uteroplacental blood flow, and fetal hypoxia (Buckley, 2015).

Educational protocols, such as the midwife-led psycho-education intervention known as **BELIEF: Birth Emotions Looking to Improve Expectant Fear,** have shown to lower the level of fear, increased ability for informed decision-making, less depressive symptoms, and improved health and obstetric outcomes. Key elements of the BELIEF system include, but are not limited to, a therapeutic relationship between the midwife and the client, support for expression of feelings, clarify misunderstandings and answer questions, enhance social support, and reinforce positive approaches to coping (Schwartz et al., 2015). These elements are not unlike traditional childbirth education classes.

Knitted Uterus

For decades, birth educators have used the knitted uterus as a model when teaching anatomy and physiology (See Diagram 3.2). It is a helpful tool to show contractions, dilation, effacement, and even cardinal movements. It can also be used to show the location of the fundus and the cervix.

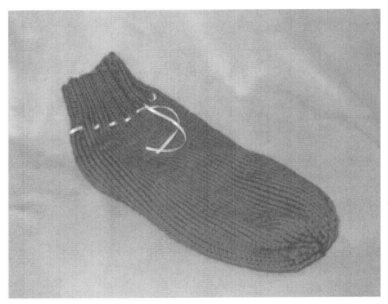

Diagram 3.2
Purchased knitted uterus

A winter knitted hat can also be used as a uterus. Select a larger-sized knitted hat, preferably without printing, logos, or pom-poms. To create a natural looking and stretchy cervix, weave elastic thread into the hat approximately one inch from the opening. Continue threading until a complete circle has been made. Make another circle with elastic 1/2 inch from the opening. Tie off the thread by pulling taut enough so the cervix is closed, but can stretch open to approximately ten centimeters. Dolls, softballs, or plastic softball-sized balls can be used to simulate the baby's head.

Pelvic "Ring"

While teaching about the importance of movement during labor, often an educator will use a model of a pelvis. She will demonstrate how it opens wider front to back with the walking motion, while opening side-to-side for movements, such as squatting or lunging.

The demonstration we call the "pelvic ring" is another method for teaching about movement during labor. You will need to wear a snug ring on one of your fingers. If you wear a wedding band, that will do just fine. The ring represents the pelvis and the finger represents the baby. Try to remove the ring simply by pulling it straight over your knuckle. This may cause pain and swelling, but eventually, you can remove the ring.

In labor, when the woman does not move throughout labor, the baby has a more difficult time getting through the pelvis, just as it is difficult to remove the ring with little movement. Then demonstrate that by wiggling the ring in a rocking motion, the ring is able to easily slip over the knuckle and be removed. Likewise, the more the mom moves her pelvis during labor, the easier it will be for the baby to inch down and through the pelvic bones.

The "pelvic ring" concept is easy to grasp for the learner. Do not be surprised if you notice the class members react to this demonstration with a greater understanding of how mom and baby are both active participants in the birth process.

Weighted Baby

A baby doll is essential when teaching any childbirth class. Most importantly, the baby is needed to show newborn care and breastfeeding. Any baby doll will do for basic instruction, but if you wish to add to the discussion, you may wish to create a weighted baby. A weighted baby is a doll weighing as much as an average-sized newborn baby.

Many dolls available on the market cannot be altered with ease. Some are not hollow, or the parts do not detach, making it difficult to add the necessary weight. Craft stores often carry the parts to create a baby doll. There are kits available at some craft stores which contain a plastic head, arms, and legs. The kit also contains a torso made of fabric and comes with the necessary clips to attach the torso to the other body parts.

To make the weighted baby with the complete kit, purchase sand or aquarium gravel and some cotton stuffing (cotton balls work well). Have a scale nearby to make sure the stuffed baby weighs approximately 7.5 pounds. Fill the legs with the sand or gravel first and attach them to the torso. Then fill the arms and attach them to the torso. Fill the head with a combination of gravel and stuffing. Put the unfinished doll plus the head on the scale and fill the torso with a combination of gravel and stuffing until the total is 7.5 pounds. Once the correct amount of filling is added, attach the head to the baby doll.

The doll can be used to teach expectant parents about positioning during breastfeeding, and you can use it to teach a sibling class about how heavy a newborn baby feels. The weighted baby is also effective for use in the Backpack Pregnant Belly (see following description).

Backpack Pregnant Belly

Most educators have heard or seen the pregnancy simulator, which allows the father to experience some of the sensations of pregnancy. He wears it on his front to look and feel like a pregnant woman. A pregnancy simulator can be a fun addition to any class. Pregnancy simulators can be professionally made with weights put in particular places to add pressure to the bladder, restrict breathing, and even add fetal movement sensations.

To make a much more simplistic pregnancy simulator that mimics the weight increase during pregnancy, and allows the father to empathize with the expectant mom, follow the directions below.

Items Needed:

- Backpack

- 25-30 lbs. of aquarium gravel

- 8 one-gallon size plastic re-sealable bags—labeled

As an added visual, choose aquarium gravel in a multitude of corresponding colors. Fill each plastic bag with the following amounts and label:

- 1 lb. Placenta

- 7.5 lbs. Baby (can use the weighted baby instead)

- 1 lb. Breasts

- 2.5 lbs. Blood

- 6 lbs. Tissue

- 2 lbs. Amniotic fluid

- 5 lbs. Fat

- 2 lbs. Uterus

Place the empty backpack on the partner's chest, having him or her insert his orher arms through the shoulder straps. While discussing the weight increase an expectant woman has, start adding the filled plastic bags one by one into the backpack. Once full, invite the partner to wear the backpack for a portion or all of the class. You can also instruct the partner to try to tie shoes, walk up and down stairs, and to get up from sitting on the floor. He or she will soon have a greater appreciation for what pregnant women must endure.

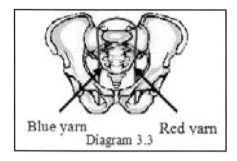

Blue yarn   Red yarn
Diagram 3.3

Yarn Vena Cava

One way to show the importance of proper positioning is to use yarn and a model of a pelvis. Take three pieces of blue yarn, each 12 inches in length, and braid them together. Do the same for three pieces of red yarn. Sew the two braided pieces together to form one 24-inch rope. Loop the rope over the top of the pelvic model, allowing the two ends of the rope to hang through the pelvic inlet (See Diagram 3.3).

With the completed rope and pelvic model, you are able to demonstrate that the arteries and veins (the *vena cava*) are less inhibited when the woman assumes an upright position. It helps to also include a fetal model in this demonstration. When the pelvis is in the supine position, the weight of the baby causes the vena cava to be somewhat compressed. This can cause less oxygen flow to and from the baby.

The Tale of the Balloon and the Ping-Pong Ball

There are so many ways to teach about labor and birth by using just two simple, inexpensive items: a balloon and a ping-pong ball. You can choose a typical 12″ balloon that is dark red to represent the uterus. Insert the ping-pong ball into the balloon. This can be somewhat tricky. The best way is to insert your index and middle fingers of both hands into the opening of the balloon. Carefully scrunch down the neck while opening it wide. The idea is to get to the main part of the balloon while having very little neck. When the balloon is opened to the center, have someone else push the ping-pong ball into the opening. If no one else is available to assist you, simply use a spare finger or two to push the ball into the balloon while other fingers keep the neck open.

Once the ball is in the balloon, blow air into the balloon until the balloon is about 6 inches in diameter. It is important to not over-inflate the balloon because too much air will make the demonstration too long to perform. Hold the balloon with the neck-side down, tugging on the neck gently while the ping-pong ball settles into the neck area, blocking the escape of air. You are now ready to begin demonstrations with this model.

Teaching Anatomy

The main body of the balloon represents the uterus while the neck of the balloon represents the uneffaced cervix. The ping-pong ball symbolizes the baby's head in the inside part of the cervix. The air in the balloon acts like the amniotic fluid.

Teaching Rupture of Membranes

A difficult subject for many expectant moms to un-der-stand is when membranes rupture, water can still leak throughout labor. You can use this model to dis-cuss the physiology of the rupturing of membranes. The baby's head makes a "cork" in the cervix, limiting the amount of fluid able to escape. When the ping-pong ball settles into the neck of the balloon, air does not escape. If the ping-pong ball dislodges from move-ment, air can leak out just as amniotic fluid can leak from around the baby's head.

Teaching Braxton-Hicks vs. True Labor Contractions

In order to teach this subject, pick up the prepared balloon model with both hands. To demonstrate Brax-ton-Hicks contractions, place both hands around the center section of the balloon and squeeze rhythmically.

Note the cervix of the model does not efface or dilate and the ball does not advance. Then place your hands on the top, or fundus, part of the balloon. Squeeze rhythmically and notice how the ping-pong ball advances, leading to effacement and eventual dilation.

Teaching Effacement and Dilatation

In the demonstration above, note how squeezing on the top part of the balloon actually causes the "cervix" to thin and open. You can show how contractions originate at the fundus of the uterus, pulling the cervix around the presenting part. The class can see how the cervix must thin out before it opens. They can also see that it takes time to dilate the cervix to complete.

Balloon and Placenta Previa

Often, expectant mothers will be told a previously low-lying placenta has "moved," and is no longer considered placenta previa. A study of anatomy and physiology shows upon implantation, the embryo develops a vascular system as a means of obtaining nutrients and eliminating waste products, by establishing an efficient interface (placenta) between its vascular system and that of its mother. Therefore, the placenta cannot actually move. To illustrate this phenomenon, draw a dime-sized dot with a permanent marker on a deflated balloon. This dot represents the newly implanted placenta. Inflate the balloon. As the balloon inflates (representing embryonic growth), the dot created by the marker appears to move. This "movement" of the dot can now be attributed to the expansion of the balloon walls with air. Similarly, as the uterus expands, the placenta appears to move.

Rubber Band for Elasticity of the Vaginal Wall

Many pregnant women and their partners have a difficult time understanding how something as large as a baby's head will fit through a canal so comparatively small. By using a size 64 rubber band, you can show how elastic the vaginal wall really can be. A relaxed rubber band symbolizes the vaginal wall at rest. It appears as if it is solid and not stretchy. Then stretch the rubber band, showing its elasticity. Similarly, the vaginal wall is made up of stretchy fibers that allow the walls to conform to the baby's head moving through it.

Elastic Bandage Perineum

Did you ever wonder how to demonstrate perineal massage effectively? One non-threatening method is to make a perineal model from a six inch diameter embroidery hoop and two 10-inch-long by 4-inch-wide pieces of elastic bandage material. Lay the two lengths of elastic bandage material (see Diagram 3.4) so they come together at the mid-point of the smaller circle of the embroidery hoop. Then lay the larger circle of the hoop over the bandage material and push until it securely fits.

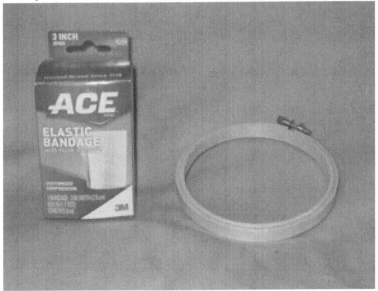

Diagram 3.4

Humorous Anatomy Cartoons

Humor can be an excellent way to capture the attention of students. There are really only two types of humor: appropriate and inappropriate. Any humor intended to divide people, belittle or ridicule, discriminate or stereotype, encourage negativity, or be at another person's expense is inappropriate. Inappropriate humor is offensive. Keep the humor on the conservative side to maintain balance and control.

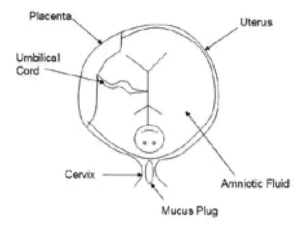

Diagram 3.5 By *Perinatal Education Associates, Inc.*

One way in which humor is often used effectively is within anecdotal illustrations. These illustrations can be simple or complex but will help to lighten the mood and foster learning. When discussing anatomy and physiology, it may be helpful to "draw" a uterus,

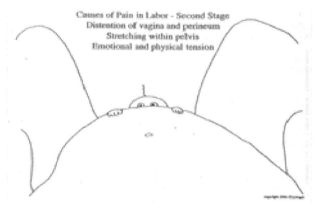

Diagram 3.7

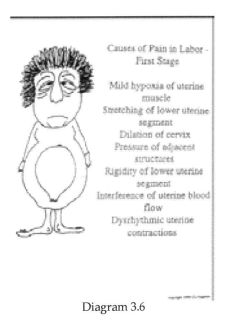

Diagram 3.6

placenta, and baby rather than show a detailed chart. Regardless of your talents as an artist, your point will get across!

This is an example of how you may actually draw a diagram of the anatomy (See Diagram 3.5). You can create a handout similar to this or simply draw this freestyle on a white-board, newsprint paper, or a chalk-board.

The following are a couple more examples of cartoons used to make light of concepts which can be anxiety producing for some individuals (See Diagrams 3.6 and 3.7).

Diet Diary

Teaching nutrition is vital, regardless of gestational age. The old phrase "eating for two" was meant to imply expectant mothers need to increase their calories, protein, vitamins, minerals, and water intake during pregnancy. It was not meant to give *carte blanche* for women to eat for two adults. Expectant mothers should have a diet that includes:

- Sufficient calories to gain weight and sustain the growing child

- An assortment of foods recommended in the *My Plate for Pregnancy* (www.choosemyplate. gov/mypryamidmoms)

- Sufficient fluid intake (approximately 64 fl oz) daily

- High-fiber foods to help prevent constipation

- Salting food to taste

- No alcohol, tobacco, or recreational pharmaceuticals

Just as no two pregnancies are going to be the same, no two women have exactly the same need for calories. Generally speaking, experts recommend an additional 300 calories in addition to a pre-pregnant caloric intake. That does not, however, mean two or three chocolate chip cookies will supply the additional 300 calories! All calories should include a variety of foods recommended in the *My Plate in Pregnancy*. However, it is important to note that pregnant women should increase their protein intake from approximately 45 grams daily to between 75 and 100 grams.

If teaching nutrition in the evening, ask the expectant mothers to write down everything they ate and drank so far that day (See Diagram 3.8). If teaching earlier in the day, ask them to write down everything they ate and drank from yesterday. Enlist the partners to assist the mothers in calculating the grams of protein. A protein counting sheet (Doula Office™ Version 2.2, 2014), and also in the class manual, *The Family Way*, by authors Debby Amis and Jeanne Green, may be helpful as a handout (Amis & Green, 2014). Expectant parents may see from the diet diary where improvement can be made.

Diet Diary

Meal:

Name of Food Item	Food Group	Serving Size	Grams of Protein

Meal:

Name of Food Item	Food Group	Serving Size	Grams of Protein

Meal:

Name of Food Item	Food Group	Serving Size	Grams of Protein

Meal:

Name of Food Item	Food Group	Serving Size	Grams of Protein

Total gram of protein today _____

Diagram 3.8

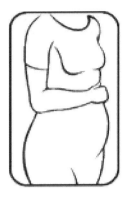

Chapter 4
The Labor Process

Tell me and I forget. Show me and I remember. Involve me and I understand.

—Chinese proverb

First Stage of Labor

Stage One of labor encompasses all of the dilation and effacement phases. Therefore, it can be considered key to the preparation for birth. When discussing this important stage, you will want to be sure to use a wide variety of teaching strategies to meet all the needs of the learners. This is definitely information you will want your students to learn and to fully understand. Combining lecture with models, acronyms, charts, handouts, hands-on activities, and more will ensure a solid knowledgebase for your clients.

Arguably, some of the most important topics to discuss about the First Stage of labor are breathing and relaxation. Proper breathing techniques and relaxation of the body can so greatly influence the labor patterns and a woman's perception of her labor that mastery becomes essential. You should be sure to reinforce these two topics throughout the course of your instruction on birth.

Breathing for Labor

There are many methods of childbirth education. Each seems to have a recommended pattern or style of breathing to be taught in the classes. Many workers and researchers in the perinatal field believe it is not so much *how* a woman breathes during labor, but that she *is* breathing. Breathing healthy and vital breaths will oxygenate the woman's body and, in turn, provide oxygen to the baby (Lothian & DeVries, 2010).

Breathing too quickly often leads directly to breathing unequally. Breathing unequally, where the intake of air is not equal to the exhale of air, often creates *hyperventilation*. Hyperventilation, too much oxygen and not enough carbon dioxide, leads to symptoms, such as dizziness, tingling of hands and lips, and "spots before your eyes." To remedy this quickly, the mother (or whomever is hyperventilating) can cup their hands over their nose and mouth and breathe in and out until the symptoms go away.

Slow, rhythmical breathing is used in many relaxation techniques, including yoga. One method to ensure those you teach have slow rhythmical breathing, with inhales equal to exhales, is to count verbally or non-verbally. When the contraction begins, many childbirth methods suggest taking a large introductory breath to signal the contraction is beginning.

After this breath, the laboring woman's support person can count "in-2-3-4 and out-2-3-4." During this counting, the laboring woman can visualize her lungs being divided into fourths, and with each number verbalized, one more fourth of her lungs are either filled with air ("in-2-3-4") or emptied of air ("out-2-3-4"). This reduces the possibility of unequal breathing, too rapid breathing, and increases focusing on external forces.

Researchers worldwide find a reduction in the respiratory rate from the normal range of 14 to 20 breaths per minute to a more therapeutic range of 10 or less breaths per minute can increase relaxation and lower blood pressure (Grossman, 2001).

Second Stage of Labor: Pushing

Renewed energy and enthusiasm typically occur during the Second Stage of labor (Littleton-Gibbs & Engebretson, 2013; Charles, 1978). It is Mother Nature's way of helping laboring mothers get through the final time before the birth of their baby. However, some mothers feel ready to push before their cervix is ready. This urge to push, or fetal ejection reflex (Kitzinger, 2011) is thought to be created by the presence of the baby's body in the birth canal, uterine contractions or surges, increased abdominal pressure, and the activation of sensory nerves carrying all of these messages to the mother's brain (Odent, 2000; Simkin et al., 2010; Simpson, 2006). This reflex cues a higher secretion of oxytocin by the pituitary gland, thus enhancing the urge.

Modern medicine is split over whether to allow women to push on demand, or to "labor down," which is to delay pushing (Avery, 2013; DiFranco & Curl, n.d.; Frey et al., 2012). Many feel that pushing on an undilated cervix will cause the cervix to swell. Therefore, when the woman feels the urge to push, and her caregiver has not given her the okay to push, repeatedly puffing air in and out as if she is blowing out a candle may help her to gain control during this difficult time, and may allow the cervix to dilate without swelling.

Regular and rhythmical breathing during pushing allows a mother to push longer while maintaining good oxygen flow to the baby and reducing fatigue. It has been suggested that avoidance of Valsalva's Maneuver (named after Italian anatomist Antonio Maria Valsalva; 1666-1723), or "Purple Pushing," can allow for a more relaxed pushing stage with minimal risk of fetal hypoxia. When the mother's breath is held for six clock seconds or longer, there is a significant metabolic scenario that takes place, as indicated in the diagram (See Diagram 4.1). Studies indicate that the mean umbilical artery pH is lower with women who "purple pushed," thus producing depressed Apgar scores (Frey et al., 2013; Prins et al., 2011). It can be said the placenta is a volume-dependent organ and changes in maternal blood volume have a significant effect on placental blood flow to the fetus.

Slow-Exhalation Pushing

Working with the urge to push and producing a push that is slow and easy, slow exhalation pushing is similar to blowing up a new balloon. During a contraction, a mother inhales and exhales slowly through pursed lips in much the same way as if she were blowing up a balloon. This is often preferred to breath holding when the baby indicates, via an electronic fetal heart monitor, he or she may not be tolerating the Second Stage well. This may also be preferred when the mother and caregiver are trying to avoid an episiotomy, since the push from Slow Exhalation Pushing is so gentle.

Spontaneous Pushing

The urge to push can be a relentless urge to push— it is nearly involuntary. To push spontaneously, many women find holding their breath during pushing increases the intensity and strength of the push. Remember, it is important to come up for air! Spontaneous pushing is most often used effectively by women who are truly in-tune with their body and respond to the overwhelming urges. No one tells them how to push or when to push. It just comes naturally.

Unfortunately, if a woman is fighting this stage of labor, not working in harmony with her body, and using this method, she may not push effectively and may hold her breath for too long. Also, this method would not be wise for a mother who is medicated and cannot feel the urge to push from the onset of the contraction.

Directed Pushing

Directed Pushing is the most commonly used type of pushing in the United States. During a contraction,

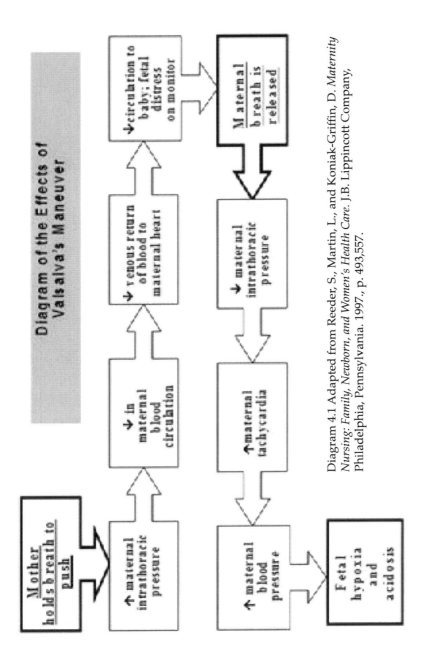

Diagram 4.1 Adapted from Reeder, S., Martin, L., and Koniak-Griffin, D. *Maternity Nursing: Family, Newborn, and Women's Health Care.* J.B. Lippincott Company, Philadelphia, Pennsylvania. 1997., p. 493,557.

a mother inhales and holds her breath while a support person counts a quick count of ten. This is not ten actual seconds, but six clock seconds. As stated previously, if a woman holds her breath for longer than six clock seconds, she can initiate Valsalva's Maneuver.

However, for clarity at a time when mothers do not process information well, a count of 10 is helpful to her. At the end of the count of 10, she exhales and inhales rapidly again, holding for another count of 10. This cycle is repeated until the contraction goes away. Usually, a woman would go through three to four series of counting to 10 per contraction.

The following teaching tips are other ways to teach about breathing and positioning for the pushing stage of labor. They appeal to the visual learners of your group and make teaching this subject more entertaining for you.

Ways to Teach Dilation and Effacement

There are suitable charts and models on the market today showing the various measurements of dilatation from one to ten centimeters. Models and charts range in price from free to hundreds of dollars (see ICEA, Perinatal Education Associates, and Childbirth Graphics).

Dilatation can also be shown by taking a piece of paper or poster board and a compass. Draw perfect circles ranging in size from one to ten centimeters diameter.

Another excellent way of teaching this sometimes dry subject is to use food items to measure dilation. The following items work well.

1 cm = 1 Cheerio or similar cereal

3 cm = diameter of a banana

7 cm = diameter of an apple

10cm = diameter of a bagel or grapefruit

Using food items with good nutritional value serves not only the purpose of this demonstration, but also provides an opportunity to promote positive eating habits. Encourage your students to choose these types of foods as possible snack items.

Food for Thoughts

Inevitably, you will have to teach people who tend to be on the quiet side. They may have ideas and questions, but need a little enticing to speak up. A great way to encourage participation is to entice them with food. Buy a bag of individually wrapped healthy snacks and offer a snack to everyone who asks a question or otherwise responds to your requests for participation. You can have even more fun with this by tossing the snack to them. Undoubtedly, as a result of this exercise you will have more participation than you can imagine.

Funnels

Funnels are an interesting way to show how labors progress at different rates, yet still lead to the same result: birth. Begin by collecting a variety of funnels from local automotive stores. Some are quite small at the top and have a long neck, others are large at the top and have a short neck. Be creative with the funnels you select.

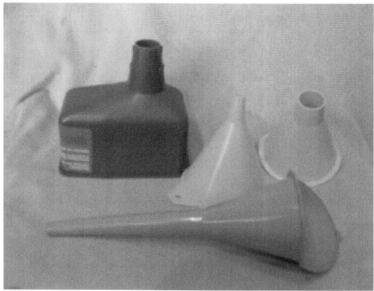

Diagram 4.2

Explain the correlation between the funnels and labor. Just as Diagram 4.2 shows, the funnel's opening begins far apart and gradually gets narrower or closer together, so do contractions. Some funnels have a very small cup that would symbolize a short labor while others show the opposite. The neck of the funnel symbolizes the pushing stage. Some have a very short neck, indicating a fast pushing stage, while others have a very long neck, signifying a long pushing stage.

Have fun with this demonstration. You may even find an enormous funnel and call it the "birth from you-know-where!" Just as these funnels, regardless of their size or shape, are still funnels, labor, no matter how short or long the stages, is still normal and serves the purpose of ushering in a new life.

Toolbox for Labor Support

When introducing class content, you can use the analogy of a toolbox. Tell the class all of the things they will learn are tools with which they can fill their toolbox. In labor, it will be good when we have a particular tool handy, if needed. They may find that they do not use all of them, but they will be glad to be able to choose what is helpful. Talk about how having the right tool really helps make the job easier. In other words, it is hard to use a flathead screwdriver when what you need is a Phillips head. Dads seem to really understand this toolbox analogy. Keep a small tool-box handy, and then write (or have them take turns writing) various tools on small pieces of paper as you discuss things, such as massage, music, relaxation, lip balm, birth ball, etc.

Rather than simply using words on a piece of paper, you can actually use items in the toolbox. For example, include a massager or two, lip balm, honey stick, sour lollipop, breath mints, CDs or iPod playlist, aromatherapy, rice sock, money for vending machines, cellphone charger, stopwatch, and whatever else you think would be good tools for labor. Lists can also be found in class manuals, such as *The Family Way* or *The Gift of Motherhood* (Customized Communications Inc.).

You can then use this toolbox later when you do a "labor rehearsal" (See Chapter 5). Read various scenarios and ask them to pick something from the toolbox, and tell them why it may be a good tool or option in the given situation.

Anatomy Teaching Tee or Apron

They say a picture is worth a thousand words. This can be a fun and eye-catching way of teaching anatomy and physiology of birth. The shirt or apron has a full color illustration of intrauterine life drawn on the material. The illustration is designed to simulate the position of the uterus and can give a realistic view of where and how the baby is positioned. This may be an affordable alternative for those who teach and cannot afford charts or videos.

Acronyms to Enhance Information Retention

Acronyms are an easy way to help expectant parents remember tips for labor and birth. The important thing is to be creative and have fun with the acronyms you use. Make them into handouts with coordinating graphics for maximum effectiveness.

P.U.R.R. or *Position, Urination, Relax, Recheck* breathing is a short way to double check on comfort measures. Quick, easy, and hits the important points.

P.U.S.H. or *Perineums Under Stress Hurt* can help them to avoid stretching the perineal tissue tight prior to crowning. The shiny, over-stretched tissue is not pliable and is ready to tear. This is the cause of many episiotomy extension tears.

T.A.C.O. (or C.O.A.T.) is a method of remembering the characteristics of the amniotic fluid if or when membranes should rupture: *Time, Amount, Color, and Odor.*

B.R.A.N.D. is a quick way to recall the aspects of informed consent: *Benefits, Risks, Alternatives, Nothing, Decide.* You can also use **B.R.A.I.N.:** *Benefits, Risks, Alternatives, Instincts, and Now* decide.

E.M.P.O.W.E.R. B.I.R.T.H.S.™ can help not only the expectant mother, but also the partner remember some important aspects of labor support. Explain the acronym as follows:

E – Encouragement. Encouragement is at the top of the list because without support, labor and delivery can be extremely challenging. Constant praise, encouragement, love, companionship, caring, and empowerment is needed to have a wonderful birth experience. Often, we look only to the physical side of birth as we anticipate labor. However, what is more important is to examine the emotional needs of the woman, because those emotions can make labor go smoothly, slowly, or stop a labor altogether. The rule: NEVER say anything negative to a laboring woman. Always stay positive and reassuring.

M – Massage. The use of touch can dramatically alter the mother's perception of pain. Touch doesn't take the pain away, but it can make it more bearable. Just think of how you would respond if you accidentally kicked a table; you would instinctively rub your foot. The mechanism is called the Gate Control Theory, which states that since the touch nerve fibers in your body are larger than the pain fibers, the touch signal gets to the brain faster, allowing the pain sensation to be minimized.

P – Position. Throughout labor, it is vitally important for the mother to change her position every 30 to

45 minutes. The descent of the baby is aided greatly by the mom's movement of the pelvis. Excellent positions are walking, squatting, slow-dancing, lunging, sitting on a birth ball, pelvic rocking, and leaning over.

O - Open Mind. Flexibility is the key to working through the birth experience. Having goals are wonderful, but it is important to remember to allow the body to work with the labor, and to keep an open mind as to options and choices along the way.

W – Walking. Although this is mentioned in "Positions" (above), it is wise to emphasize its importance. Walking throughout the pregnancy and into the labor really can help prepare mom's body for the physical side of birth. It allows excellent pelvic mobility, which is necessary for fetal descent. Also, walking seems to ease the pain of labor for most women.

E - Empty Bladder. As with each position change, the mother should try to empty her bladder every 30 to 45 minutes to open the pathway for the baby. Over and over again, birth is delayed for minutes, and even hours, as a result of a full bladder. If the mother is not able to urinate for more than a couple of hours, then straight catheterization may be warranted.

R – Refreshments. The mother needs to maintain fluid and nutritional levels during the labor process. Depriving a mother of nutrients and fluids greatly reduces her stamina for labor. Birth is an intense workout for the body. Without energy, the body cannot work efficiently. The mother should take in fluids, such as water, juices, or clear sport drinks throughout the early and active phase of labor, and as needed in transition and pushing. Nutrients can be obtained by eating easily digested foods in early labor to active labor (i.e., broth, yogurt, JELL-O,® crackers, dry toast, and plain baked potato).

B – Breathing. Encourage the mother to explore her breathing technique options to see what best fits her needs. Regardless of the method, what she needs to remember is to BREATHE—not to hold her breath. When we are faced with pain or stress, we have a tendency to hold our breath. In labor, the body and baby need that oxygen throughout the contractions. KEEP BREATHING.

I – Imagery. Some women really respond well to guided imagery. Explore this option if this is something you think might help the mother to relax. Imagery is simply allowing the mind to wander to a peaceful place (beach, mountains, green grassy meadow, etc.) and taking in all the sites, smells, sounds, and feelings of that special place.

R – Relaxation. Maintaining a calm and relaxed state is the most important tool for labor. The more deeply we can relax, the more efficiently our body can work and the less pain we feel. If you think about it, one of the reasons why medications are given in labor is to relax the body.

T – Trust. The woman's body is designed to give birth normally and naturally. For the great majority of women, if they trust in their body and abilities and have the necessary support, they can birth naturally.

H – Honor the Process. Never forget the reason for the labor experience; the ushering in of a new life. Take this opportunity to realize the miracle of birth. This birth experience will remain in their hearts for a lifetime and affect each person with whom they share their story. Always remember to respect and honor the process.

S – Surroundings. Set the appropriate mood by altering the lighting, sounds, and smells in the room. If you wish to evoke a calm, relaxed state, then try dimming the lights, lighting candles (not in a hospital room, though), putting on soft music, and perhaps using aromatherapy.

Lifesavers® Dilation and Effacement

A Lifesavers® candy can effectively demonstrate labor takes time to progress. The candy is also effective in teaching about effacement and dilation. Purchase a roll of Lifesavers®, give one to each class participant, and tell them not to bite it! Over time, the candy will melt away (labor), thin (efface), and the hole will open (dilate).

Turtleneck Effacement and Dilation

Cervical dilation and effacement can easily be de-mon-strated by pulling a turtleneck over your head. Think of the neck of the turtleneck as the cervix. When first placing the shirt over the head, the neck of the turtleneck is long (uneffaced). As you slowly pull the shirt over your head, the neck begins to efface. Notice it effaces before opening (dilating). As the neck becomes completely effaced, it begins to dilate at a faster pace until it is complete. Complete is the point where the neck is making a headband around your head, and the rest of the head slides through easily.

Balloons for Slow Exhalation Pushing and Muscle Isolation

New balloons are a fun way to help expectant mothers isolate the abdominal muscles needed for pushing during the Second Stage of labor. When teaching about pushing, have the expectant mothers assume a preferred pushing position, such as squatting, or using gravity. Give her a balloon and have her blow into it. She may feel a slight bulging of the perineal muscles as she blows into the balloon. Explain to her the involvement of these muscles in pushing. (*Be aware of latex balloons and potential latex allergies.*)

Using the balloon demonstrates exhaling can occur without release of tension by the abdominal muscles. Care providers often desire a constant push by the laboring woman in conjunction with the contraction to make the most of the contraction. With adequate practice, the expectant mother can learn to keep the pressure during the push, while still allowing proper oxygenation of the uterus and baby. Some mothers have found this exercise so helpful, they have added balloons to their labor goodie bags. This exercise may also be helpful for mothers with epidural anesthesia.

Birthday Candle + Feather Blowing

Often expectant parents hear stories about the difficulties of avoiding a premature urge to push. Each woman who has experienced this premature urge to push knows how difficult it is to not push. However, until the cervix is complete, it is important not to push with force. That way, it is less likely that the cervix will swell or tear from the premature pushing.

To aid in the avoidance of pushing, the laboring mom can lift her chin upwards and blow. Blowing upwards minimizes the force of any involuntary pushing. She can also pretend she is blowing out the baby's birthday candle, and the candle is one of those trick candles that keeps relighting. Another option is to imagine that there is a feather floating above and the laboring woman must keep it afloat. She gives gentle puffs to keep the feather from falling to the ground.

Vent Hose + Tennis Ball

Much has been written about the benefits of upright position-ing during labor and birth. Grav-ity helps with effacement and di-lation of the cervix by applying pressure on the cervix, enabling the stretching and breaking of the connective tissue bands in the cer-vix. Stretching and breaking of these bands facilitates the release of the prostaglandin hormone which, in turn, softens the cervix and makes it more receptive to the force of the gravity.

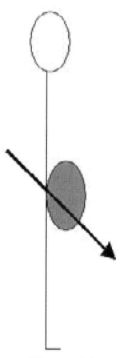

Diagram 4.4

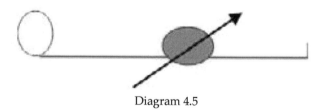

Diagram 4.5

Assuming an upright position also changes the *drive angle* of the baby in comparison to the mother's pelvis. When the drive angle is pointed downward, the mother has to exert much less effort when pushing the baby out (See Diagram 4.4).

When the drive angle is pointed upward, the mother has to fight gravity and exert much more effort when pushing (See Diagram 4.5).

When teaching this concept, you can use an effective technique to demonstrate the benefits of the upright position for birth.

Use a piece of flexible dryer vent hose (or flexible hose/tunnel purchased at a pet store for hamsters) and a tennis ball. When one end of the hose is positioned up and the other (exit) is down, gravity allows for a more rapid descent of the tennis ball. When the dryer hose is lying flat, or when the exit is pointing upward, more power from the mother is needed for expulsion.

PVC Piping

PVC piping also works for demonstrating the need for upright positioning and the benefits for labor and birth. Substitute a 10 centimeter diameter piece of PVC piping with a 45 degree angle bend for the flexible dryer vent hose. Just as with the dryer vent hose demonstration, the PVC piping shows the J-shaped angle the baby will need to travel to get down and under the pubic bone.

When the PVC piping is angled upward, it requires energy to push the ball through the piping to the other side. When the PVC piping is angled downward, as if the expectant mother is leaning over a birthing ball and the pelvic outlet is angled downward, the ball will freely travel through the PVC piping.

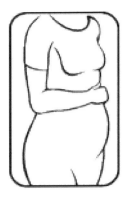

Chapter 5
Teaching Comfort Measures

The wisdom and compassion a woman can intuitively experience in childbirth can make her a source of healing and understanding for other women.

—Stephen Gaskin

Non-pharmacologic pain relief therapies are ways to decrease pain without the use of medication or pharmacology, hence the name *non–pharmacologic*. These therapies, while used in other facets of health care, can be very effective during labor and birth. Additionally, these therapies are non-invasive and appear to be safe for mother and baby.

In most cultures, pain is an indicator that something is wrong. However, pain during childbirth actually tells the expectant mother and her partner where she is in her labor. If the chart below is an accurate indicator, one can estimate by emotional changes how far along (in centimeters of dilation and percent of effacement) the mother is in the Phases of Stage One labor.

Stages of Labor	Dilation (cms)	Efface- ment (%)	Dura- tion/fre- quency	Emotional Cues
Stage 1				
Early Phase	0-3 cm	Varies	30 sec/30 mins	Happy, excited
Active Phase	4-6 cm	Varies (~30%)	60 sec/3-5 mins	Focused, making an effort
Transition Phase	7-10 cms	100%	90 sec/1-2 mins	Struggling, painful
Stage 2				
Pushing & Birth of the Baby			60 sec/3-5 mins	Spontaneous bearing down; focused; determined

Stage 3				
Birth of Placenta			Mild	
Stage 4				
The Gold-en Hour after Birth			Mild as invo-lution occurs	Joy, elation, curious about baby

A childbirth education class is particularly helpful in giving expectant parents information about using both non-pharmacologic pain relief, as well as medication for pain relief.

With the knowledge of anatomy/physiology and pain, class members will also begin brainstorming possible ways to reduce the perception of pain based on their previous experiences. A basic question to ask would be, "how do you self-soothe?" To lead the group in a discussion, ask what they do when they stub their toe. Most often, other than muttering some colorful language, people will rub their toe. While they are rubbing their toe, the pain seems to fade. This is due to the Gate Control Theory.

First published in 1965, Melzack and Wall introduced a new pain mechanism theory (Melzack & Wall, 1965). The perception of pain is a dance between the Central Nervous System (brain and spinal cord) and the Peripheral Nervous System (branching nerves in the torso and extremities). Since human-touch fibers are larger and the perception of touch moves faster, the sensation of touch will reach the brain first or overload it. The human-pain fibers are smaller, and the perception of touch moves slower. Therefore, non-pharmacologic pain relief methods, such as massage, heat, and cold, laboring in the water will stimulate the touch fibers and send a more pleasurable message than pain to the brain. The brain does sense some pain, and when this happens, morphine-like substances called endorphins are produced to help handle the pain sensations.

To demonstrate the many choices of non-pharmacologic pain relief available to expectant mothers and their partners, charts or handouts like the one below are beneficial. From the Listening to Mothers II survey (Declercq et al., 2006), only 50% of those surveyed used structured breathing techniques, and breathing techniques were rated as least helpful. However, the non-pharmacologic pain relief techniques that were rated most helpful were hydrotherapy, effleurage/massage, sitting on the birth ball, and showering.

Heat and Cold Therapy

Applications of heat and cold are the most common inexpensive, non-invasive pain relief methods. In general, heat relaxes and cold numbs. Depending on the need of the laboring mother, heat and cold therapy positively influences the perception of pain. Heat relaxes tissues and opens up blood vessels, increasing blood flow and hence, supplying more oxygen (Littleton-Gibbs & Engebretson, 2013).

Nutrition and Hydration

A discussion of Nutrition/Hydration would focus around the "ice chips only" policy of some birth facilities. This has a history dating back to the 1940s and Mendelson's Syndrome, or aspiration of vomit during general anesthesia (Medelson, 1946). With labor occurring often before the administration of general anesthesia, a delay in gastric emptying is one of the major reasons why oral intake has been prohibited.

This traditional policy of restricted food and fluids has lasted over 50 years. In a 2010 Cochrane review of restricting oral fluid and food intake during labor, the reviewers found that there is no evidence of benefits or harm with low-risk women requiring general anesthesia (Sinqata et al., 2013). These reviewers also felt that women should have the autonomy and freedom to choose to eat or drink during labor. It was found that women naturally reduce oral intake as labor progresses and is more intense. However, more research is needed to examine a policy of restricted food and fluids with certain obstetrical interventions, such as regional anesthesia or oxytocin induction/augmentation. Additional research focusing on the effects of fluid and food restriction and mid-labor stall of contractions would also be helpful.

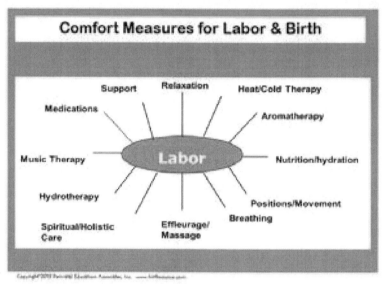

Diagram 6.1

Prior to the 1970s natural childbirth movement, pregnant women had a number of social influences on them. Pregnant women were not to travel much, maternity clothes were not very flattering, and there was very little information given to pregnant women regarding their upcoming labor and birth. Since the 1970s, wisdom from the past has been reintroduced as new techniques to help mothers have positive pregnancy outcomes.

Upright and Gravity Positive Positions and Movements

Information about the Cardinal Movements that the baby's complete during labor leads to the need for position changes during labor to facilitate those Movements. An upright position allows for an increase in the pelvic diameter and reduced direct pressure on the coccyx or tailbone. Using a variety of positions, and changing about every 20 minutes, will enhance the progress of labor by not inhibiting the Cardinal Movements.

During a comfort measures class, using demonstration/return demonstration to introduce the various positions for labor will reduce the apprehension in assuming some of the positions. Positions to introduce and practice during class include standing, swaying, slow dancing with the partner, kneeling on all fours, kneeling on all fours using a birthing ball, sitting, lunging, sitting on the birthing ball, squatting, sitting backwards on a chair, sitting on the toilet, and side-lying. Basically, any upright and gravity positive position helps to bring the baby down and out without hindrance.

In an observational cohort study done (Gizzo et al., 2014), it was found that upright, gravity-positive positions were associated with less pain, lower anesthesia rate, reduced length of labor, as well as an increase in the laboring woman's comfort and satisfaction after the birth. The researchers also cite studies that suggest that movement restriction during labor due to certain interventions (medication, electronic fetal monitoring) may in-crease the incidence of dystocia.

What is a Birthing Ball?

Birthing balls are one of the useful tools used in pregnancy and labor. A birthing ball is really a *professional* physical therapy ball. Professional physical therapy balls are widely used to promote good posture, alleviate back pain, and encourage mobility (Taavoni et al., 2011). Gyms throughout the country use these physical therapy balls in stretching exercises and workout routines. These medical-grade physical therapy balls were brought to the birthing arena because of their benefits to pregnant and birthing women. Thus, these balls obtained the name "Birthing Balls."

Birthing balls can help expectant/laboring women get into positions that are more comfortable, and can enhance labor's progress. These positions provide movement to change the position of the baby if necessary. Expectant parents may first become familiar with a birthing ball during a childbirth education class or during a tour of the facility in which they will be giving birth. Many expectant parents have even purchased their own birthing balls. It is important to point out that professional birthing balls __*are not*__ the same as the large balls seen in toy stores or discount centers. Birthing balls are now being used in many birthing centers, at home births, as well as hospitals, because of the usefulness to laboring women.

Selecting a Birthing Ball

There are many retail stores and websites that both promote and sell birthing balls of all sizes and colors. Which ball is the *right* one? How do you choose with so many sources? The birthing ball should be large enough for the expectant mother to sit on with her legs bent at a 90-degree angle. If the ball will be used for a wide variety of pregnant women, the 65 cm ball is best. Air can be added or removed to allow the ball to fit most women (5' 2" to 5'10" in height) and weight (up to 600 lbs.).

Some mothers prefer a round ball because it sits low to the ground and movement towards the front and back are minimized. This allows for greater stability, and also puts the woman in a deeper squat. It is ideal for a prolonged pushing stage. The pictures below show both the front and side views of sitting on the Peanut Ball, which provides more stability and comfort.

Birthing balls can be made of a variety of materials and have small ribbing to retard slippage. Latex is one of the most popular materials used to make birthing balls. Many expectant mothers are discovering that they are latex allergic, and it is extremely important for individuals with known *latex allergies* to avoid birthing balls made of such material. Latex-free birthing balls are readily available, and can be cleaned and maintained easily.

A major concern of those purchasing birthing balls is *sudden deflation factor*; that is, the rate at which a birthing ball will deflate after puncture with a person sitting on the ball. Many birthing balls that were previously available were made of materials that had a high sudden-deflation factor. Midwives, childbirth educators, doulas, and nurses in hospitals where birthing balls are used, now seek out birthing balls with a low sudden-deflation factor. Slow-deflating birthing balls allow for the expectant mother to get off of the deflating ball before injury can occur.

Deflation factor is different from being weight tested. Most balls sold today for laboring women are weight tested from 450 to 600 lbs. This is in drastic contrast to balls seen in toy stores that are not made of slow-deflate material, and may not have been weight tested. Always keep sharp objects away from the birthing ball to avoid unnecessary puncturing. The birthing ball may be inflated with a dual-action ball pump or an air mattress pump. It should be inflated to the point that is slightly firm, but still "gives" and it should roll easily (Livingston, 2014).

All of these factors may be of interest to the hospital or birth facility risk management department.

General Use of a Birthing Ball

In the last months of pregnancy, a pregnant woman's center of gravity changes as the baby gains weight and length. The center of gravity pulls the mother forward, making movement awkward, slow, and difficult. Additionally, the same hormones that relax the cartilage in the pelvis also relax the knees as well. This often makes it difficult to get up and down from a sitting position.

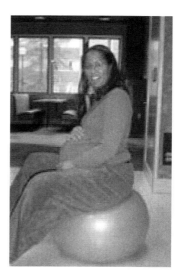

Many women find sitting on a birthing ball at home, watching television, or working on the computer easier than sitting in a chair or couch. Sitting on a birthing ball also encourages pelvic mobility, helping mothers to not feel stiff and uncomfortable while sitting.

Sitting upright in a gravity-positive position and moving on the birthing ball enhances descent of the baby through the pelvic bones, taking advantage of gravity. It allows the mother the freedom to rock her pelvis, change her position, and easily shift her weight for comfort.

The birthing ball enhances relaxation of the pelvic floor muscles, or "Kegels," by conforming to the mother's body. The ball encourages pelvic relaxation by conforming to the mother's body, similar to a water bed mattress, as it provides *perineal support* without undue pressure. Sitting on warm compresses on the birthing ball will also enhance pelvic floor relaxation.

Most hospitals today are making use of birthing balls for their patients because of the favorable benefits and results. Check availability of local birth facilities to make sure they have them in the maternity unit.

Sitting on the ball helps to position the baby or keep the baby well-aligned in the pelvis, and assist in correcting an *ascynclitic* presentation–where the baby's head is in a "crooked" position in the pelvis. Squatting helps widen the pelvic outlet to its maximum. The ball encourages rhythmic movement as the mother sways, and rocks back and forth while sitting on the ball, allowing for the baby to turn from ascynclitic, or posterior positions, to vertex.

Position changes and movement on the ball may speed up labor due to the opening of the pelvic bones. When a pregnant woman sits on a birthing ball, her pelvis opens 1 to 2 cm wider than other positions.

The birthing ball can even be used with both the external and internal electronic fetal monitoring, should monitoring become necessary. Checking with a labor nurse or doula for the hospital policy regarding the use of the birthing ball is advisable for particular situations. A labor nurse or doula may place a water-proof pad, or "chux" pad, over the ball while the mother is laboring on it. If the amniotic sac breaks or is leaking while the mother is on the birthing ball, a chux pad will help maintain cleanliness and comfort.

Positioning on the all may speed up labor through the use of gravity. The laboring mother can also use the ball to curl around, should they elect to have epidural anesthesia. Studies have shown that sitting on the birthing ball, either round or Peanut, can reduce the perception of pain experienced by the laboring woman.

When a woman is pregnant, the center of gravity is altered and she will need someone to help steady her while preparing to sit on the ball to avoid becoming off-balanced. Using the birthing ball with a "spotter," or someone to watch over the mother, such as a labor nurse or doula, is a wise option. When in the hospital setting, and there is only one labor-support person available, the ball can be forced against the end of the labor bed or some other sturdy object to steady it as the mother sits down.

Another concern when using birthing balls with expectant mothers is stability. Now, there are birthing ball bases available for purchase. These durable plastic, easy-to-clean bases steady the ball while expectant mothers sit, rock, and sway their pelvises. Ball bases are ideal for the hospital setting where only one support person is available for the expectant mother, or for home or work where the mother must sit for long periods of time. The bases, when used with the birthing ball, also allows for better posture.

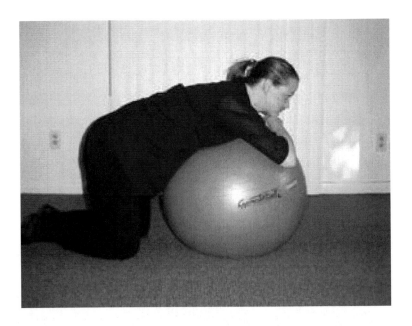

Expectant mothers often suffer from incorrect posture, which can lead to stiff shoulders and neck, backaches, leg aches, and even headaches. Birthing ball bases are an ideal alternative to chairs for expectant mothers.

To sit properly, the mother should stand with her back to the ball with feet firmly on the floor, and at least shoulder width apart. The mother should wear non-skid shoes or slippers to prevent slipping. The support person then guides the woman into the sitting position on the ball. The mother's thighs and feet should be turned in the same direction. The labor-support person can then sit in front of the mother while offering encouragement, or behind while applying massage techniques.

When the nurse, midwife, or physician has confirmed the diagnosis of posterior presentation, have the mother lean over the birthing ball while on her hands and knees. This position gives her good pelvic mobility, as well as the use of gravity to encourage the largest and heaviest part of the baby's body to rotate. As the mother's weight is totally supported by the birthing ball, she is able to stay in the hands/knees position for an extended period of time.

Normally, the mother is only able to stay in this position for a short interval, as it aggravates carpal tunnel syndrome by putting excess strain on wrists and hands. Without the birthing ball, this position is tiring, as she must support her entire body weight. Being in this position causes the baby to be cradled in the sling that the abdominal muscles form. Doing the Pelvic-Rock exercise while in this position helps to initiate the baby to turn to the favorable anterior position approximately 85% of the time.

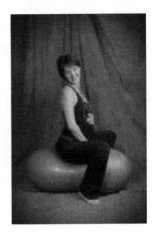

It is also easier for a support person to apply counter-pressure for the mother's back pain while the mother is in the hands and knees, or "all fours" position, and resting the weight of her body on the ball. Massage and/or counter-pressure can be easily applied with a massage tool or hands. The expectant mother also avoids over using her wrists to support her body, thus avoiding aggravating carpal tunnel syndrome (Kwan et al., 2011).

A birthing ball can also be used in a shower or bathtub for the expectant mother to sit on or lean over. If using a bathtub, be certain to wedge the ball securely between the sides of the tub. Take care so that the ball does not slip out of place. The best position for use in a tub is when the mother is in an "all-fours" position leaning over the ball.

The birthing ball can also be used in the labor tub—wedging the ball between the sides of the tub and adding a towel to the bottom of the tub reduces slippage.

If the mother will be using the ball to sit in a shower, there should be adequate support close by to assist her onto the ball and off the ball. The ball is an excellent choice for the mother who wants the benefits of hydrotherapy while enjoying the comfort of the birthing ball.

Peanut birthing balls can help expectant/laboring women get into positions that are more comfortable and can enhance labor's progress. These positions provide movement to change the position of the baby, if necessary. Some of the positions that can be used with the peanut birthing ball include The Straddle, Straddle/Lunge, laboring on all fours on the ball and knees, laboring on all fours standing, and sidelying with leg supported by the ball. Partners and helpers can use massage techniques or counter-pressure techniques to relieve back labor easily with the peanut ball. Peanut balls can also be used to increase pelvic outlet size for the turning of an asynclitic baby, or to enable the laboring mother to assume a stable and supported deep squat for early pushing or laboring down. Again, research shows that using a birthing ball reduces the laboring mother's perception of pain.

The use of the peanut birth ball has received much more attention since the 2011 study by Banner Health Hospitals in Arizona, Colorado, etc. A randomized control trial was done with over 200 expectant mothers. The peanut ball was used on women who received epidural anesthesia and could not use other proven birthing methods, such as squatting or movement using the conventional round birthing ball. Those who used the peanut ball decreased the First Stage of labor by nearly 90 minutes, and the Second Stage of labor by 23 minutes compared with a control group that did not use the ball. Further, when examining statistical data regarding cesarean section rates, the group who used the peanut ball was 13% lower than the control group who did not use the ball.

Sitting on the birth ball has also been shown to reduce assisted deliveries (forceps/vacuum), reduction in episiotomies, and fewer abnormal fetal heartrate patterns (Livingston, 2014).

Movement during labor is important and there are many benefits. Practicing the various positions in class will make them real and allow the expectant parents to feel free to use them while in labor.

Breathing

While there are limited studies regarding the use of breathing and birth outcomes, there is a myriad of studies demonstrating the use of the breath in reducing stress, anxiety, and panic. As mentioned before, stress hormones can cause uterine muscle hypoxia, interruption in utero-placental blood flow, and fetal hypoxia. They are also responsible for a slowing, or even cessation, of uterine contractions by influencing the secretion of oxytocin. Structured breathing techniques may not be totally effective on their own for non-pharmacologic pain relief. However, in conjunction with other techniques, breathing can maintain oxygenation levels for the baby and the uterus (Lothian & DeVries, 2010).

Effleurage/Massage

When Fernand Lamaze's notes were translated from French into English, the only word that was not translated was effleurage. Effleurage is a light and gentle circular stroking of an expectant woman's abdomen with fingertips; either her own or her support person's fingers. This is often done during the contraction (practice or real), along with breathing and focusing. In reference to the Gate Control Theory, performing three complex acts simultaneously allows little room for perception of pain sensations.

Aromatherapy

The use of aromatherapy and essential oils dates back nearly 5,000 years and occurs in a variety of cultures. Uses included spiritual or ritualistic purposes, cosmetic adornment, as well as therapeutic use.

French chemist, Rene-Maurice Gattefosse, founded the science of aromatherapy in the late 1920s after applying lavender oil on his own burnt hand.

While it is not fully understood how or why essential oils produce the effects that they do, one obvious way that essential oils work is through the sense of smell. This sense is incredibly powerful: according to some estimates, about 10,000 times stronger than any other sense. The "smell" receptors in your nose communicate with two structures that are embedded deep in your brain, and serve as storehouses for emotions and memories. These structures are called the amygdala and hippocampus. When essential oil molecules are inhaled, they affect these parts of the brain directly. Researchers believe that stimulation of these structures can affect our physical, emotional, and mental health.

It is also known that breathing in essential oils can affect the respiratory system. For example, certain oils from the eucalyptus plant are able to clear sinuses and prevent respiratory infections. Hence, the reason why Hall's Mentholyptus™ and Vicks™ are so popular during cold and flu season.

The reduction of stress and anxiety is one of the specific uses of aromatherapy during labor. While it is well established that maternal anxiety and stress during labor can decrease the effectiveness of contractions, increase labor duration, and also increase the likelihood of intervention, aromatherapy may be used to produce a feeling of calm and comfort by stimulation of the olfactory system. Studies have demonstrated that some of the most effective essences to be lavender oil, citrus aurantium oil (also known as neroli), rose, and peppermint (Namazi et al., 2014).

The week before introducing essential oils in class, find out if there are any attendees who have allergies to or sensitivities to essential oils. If not, a variety of high-quality, essential oils can be passed around the class. Consult with a certified aromatherapist before allowing class members to apply oils to the skin, as some oils can produce a rash or itching. To find an aromatherapist, contact the National Association of Holistic Therapy (www.naha.org). The aromatherapist will be able to provide additional information on use, contraindications, and side effects. Ingestion of essential oils has been practiced in Europe for some time, yet there is little evidence-based scientific information that ingestion of essential oils in the U.S. is safe or effective.

Music Therapy

Music sets a mood. Women who use music as a relaxation enhancer during the labor and birthing process may have lower pain and anxiety reactions than those who do not use music (Simavli et al., 2014). A landmark study from 1981 also found that music served additional functions during the birth process, including increased focus, distraction from the pain, stimulating pleasurable responses, focused breathing, and a conditioned stimulus for relaxation (Clark et al., 1981). Music Therapy Assisted Childbirth (MTAC) was developed as a result of the exploration of the use of "audio-analgesia" (sounds for discomfort relief) in the 1980s. In the MTAC Program, music therapists assist expectant parents in selecting music for birth.

Familiarity with the music through consistent practice with the music, relaxation, and breathing produces the best response during labor and birth. Childbirth educators and doulas, while not music therapists, can also help expectant parents find music that they can use for relaxation and practice.

Hydrotherapy: Water Labor and Birth

The concept of hydrotherapy use during labor is not new. The first documented water labor (and subsequent birth) occurred in 1803 in France. In 1963, Igor Charkovsky experimented with water and labor in the Soviet Union. Hydrotherapy in labor has been used in the United States for many years (ICEA Position Paper Water Labor, Water Birth, 2014).

For many women, hydrotherapy, or the use of water as a non-pharmacologic pain relief technique, is highly desirable for labor. Hydrotherapy may be in the form of a warm spray of water from the shower aimed at the lower uterine segment to relieve the stretching sensations of the ligaments and areas associated with posterior presentations. Water immersion can reduce labor pain, and is associated with fewer cesarean sections. Immersion has also been associated with shorter length of labor, reduction in the use of anesthesia, fewer vaginal/perineal lacerations, and a reduction in SUI (stress urinary incontinence) at 6 weeks postpartum (Harper et al., 2012).

Laboring in a labor tub can increase a laboring woman's pain tolerance (the duration or intensity of pain that the woman is willing to endure). The hydrostatic pressure of the water relieves some of the discomforts of the contractions. Tubs that maintain the water temperature at or around body temperature (98° F to100° F) also soothes tired and aching muscles and ligaments, furthering relaxation of the mother (Liu et al., 2014). Buoyancy [a concept discovered by Greek mathematician, Archimedes (287 to 212 BC)] in the labor tub allows for an almost weightless feeling. Women who need to move during labor to enhance progress truly benefit from the ease of movement in a labor tub. Thus, hydrotherapy may improve uterine dystocia and reduce the need for augmentation and epidural use.

Critical to any discussion of water labor and water birth is the immediate reaction of the mother to bring her baby to her chest, and the natural reaction to begin skin-to-skin contact. Annie Sprague sums it up:

> Using both qualitative and quantitative methodologies to research this topic for my thesis, it became apparent that water immersion during labor and birth was also associated with decreased rates of perineal trauma, episiotomy rates, and operative deliveries (cesarean sections, forceps or ventouse). This was coupled with increased maternal satisfaction with the experience of childbirth, when compared with births where water immersion was not used during labor and birth (Sprague, 2011).

According the late Sheila Kitzinger, in her book, *The Complete Book of Pregnancy and Childbirth (2nd Edition)*:

> Lying in warm water increases venous pressure so that veins can return blood to the heart more efficiently. It also enhances cardiac action and slows the pulse rate (Kitzinger, 2003).

Kitzinger also includes a wonderful section on "Exploring Birth Movements in Water." The photos are a must-see for those working with women and labor tubs. For communities where hydrotherapy is currently unavailable, teaching about the benefits of hydrotherapy may not change the birthing landscape today, but it does lay the groundwork for change in the future. In the study, Liu et al. compared water immersion and regional anesthesia. They found that water immersion during labor was convenient, comfortable, and had no side effects, making it nearly the ideal method of providing pain relief during labor (Liu et al., 2014).

Spiritual and Holistic Care

Tapping into the expectant parents' holistic or spiritual beliefs may greatly impact the ability of the woman to relax during labor. If the expectant parents have a spiritual foundation, acknowledging the use of traditional methods such as prayer or meditation gives "permission" to use these methods during labor and birth. Some research shows that prayer may positively influence heartrate, blood pressure, and anxiety (Beiranvand et al., 2014). A childbirth educator or doula can assist parents by brain-storming possible methods to use during labor and birth, but must refrain from inserting pressure for a particular way.

Social Support

The positive effects of social support during labor and birth are well-documented. The role of the doula, a trained labor support professional, is also well-documented in the medical literature. Drs. Marshall Klaus and John Kennell spent over 20 years researching the benefits of doula support. Those findings, as well as the findings of other researchers, show that women with labor support are 28% less likely to have a cesarean birth, 31% less likely to have their labor augmented, 9% less likely to use pain medication, and 34% less likely to rate their childbirth experience negatively (ICEA Position Paper: Role and Scope of the Birth Doula, 2014).

Having a doula come to a childbirth education class as a guest speaker can be an exciting opportunity for the class members. They can freely ask questions and explore their community options. The doula can explain that support can come from suggesting alternative positions, maintaining fluid intake, and using various non-pharmacologic pain relief techniques. It is important to point out (or for the doula to point out) that support is not limited to non-pharmacologic techniques. Doulas can be beneficial for those choosing medication or having a cesarean birth.

Relaxation

Relaxing during labor might seem to be an oxymoron. However, the benefits of relaxing during labor are many. Research demonstrates that even simple relaxation with a CD of relaxation techniques, positive affirmations, and guided imagery had significant impact on women's perception of pain indicated by the use of the Edmonton Scale (www.npcre.org/files/edmonton_symptoms_assessment_scale.pdf).

Pain has two components: threshold and tolerance. Pain threshold is the point at which an individual recognizes pain. This is a variable, as some persons do not quickly feel pain, while others sense it almost before it happens. Pain tolerance, on the other hand, is the ability of a human to withstand pain, including intensity, as soon as it is recognized. This, too, is variable, and dependent on a variety of stimulation by the external environment. In labor, pain is caused by ischemia of the uterine muscle, stretching and traction of the uterine ligaments, traction of the ovaries, pressure on the urethra, bladder, and rectum, and distention of the lower uterine segment, pelvic floor muscles, and perineum.

Dr. Grantly Dick-Read identified the now-famous "Fear-Tension-Pain Cycle" (Dick-Read, 2013). This cycle demonstrates that if a person has fear about a certain event, there is also tension in their bodies. If there is tension, the tension can amplify any pain present. This, in turn, can increase the person's fear. An increase in fear also increases tension and pain. Thus, the cycle continues and grows. However, if at some point, the cycle is broken with education and research and relaxation techniques, the amount of pain perceived by the person is reduced. According to *The Healthy Pregnancy Book* by Sears et al. (2013), tense muscles hurt more than relaxed muscles. There is a series of chemical changes that occur, which lowers the muscles pain threshold and allows for a higher perception of pain. As with any sustained pain, there is exhaustion, which also interferes with a person's ability to tolerate pain (Sears et al., 2013).

Relaxation works against stress and anxiety in the body. Dr. Herbert Benson (Benson & Klipper, 2000) identified the "relaxation response" as an opposite re-action to the "fight or flight" response. Benson found that in a deep state of relaxation, the body experiences a decrease in blood pressure, heartrate, muscle tension, and breathing. There are increased feelings of calm and being in control. Studies have shown that relax-ation techniques can reduce the perception of pain, re-duce the need for medication, and can often enhance the immune response.

Benson's stress response begins in the brain, where the amygdala interprets images and sounds as danger. In the amygdala, the image/sound event may be found to be dangerous, and a message is sent to the hypo-thalamus. The hypothalamus communicates with the entire body via the autonomic nervous system (AVS). This system influences the involuntary reactions, such as blood pressure, heartrate, and breathing. Within the AVS are the para-sympathetic nervous system and the sympathetic nervous system. The parasympathetic nervous system (PNS) promotes relaxation, calming, and evaluation of the stress event. The sympathetic nervous system (SNS) is the home of the "flight or fight" reaction–stimulating the stress hormone epinephrine, which can counterbalance the effect of oxytocin and slow or stop labor. If left in "flight or fight" mode long enough, the body also releases cortisol, which helps to maintain the "flight or fight" feeling.

Practicing relaxation techniques helps to make the relaxation response a part of a lifestyle, rather than something learned in a childbirth class. In fact, practicing for 20 minutes per day may significantly reduce cortisol levels. According to Prevention.com (www.prevention.com/mind-body/how-lower-cortisol-manage-stress), relaxation/meditation reduces cortisol by 20% using music can cut cortisol levels by 66%, and being massaged can reduce cortisol by 31%.

Relaxation instruction and practice is vital in any childbirth education class or doula visit. Effective and frequently used methods of relaxation include meditation, progressive muscle relaxation, guided visualization, and yoga nidra. Tutorials on these can be found on the following websites and apps:

Meditation

> http://stress.about.com/od/meditation/tp/Learn-How-To-Meditate.htm

> http://www.mindbodygreen.com/0-14150/how-to-meditate-in-a-minute-video-tutorial.html

Progressive Muscle Relaxation

> http://www.anxietybc.com/sites/default/
> files/MuscleRelaxation.pdf
>
> http://www.cci.health.wa.gov.au/docs/ACF-
> 3C8D.pdf

Guided Visualization

> http://www.innerhealthstudio.com/guid-
> ed-imagery-scripts.html
>
> http://www.icea.org/sites/default/
> files/09-07.pdf - see Page 4, "Guided Imagery: a
> Best Practice for Pregnancy and Childbirth" by
> Belleruth Naparstek.

Yoga Nidra

> iTunes or Android App "Simply Being" (Free)

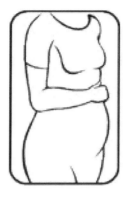

Chapter 6
Reviews and Rehearsals

Good teaching is one-fourth preparation and three-fourths theater.

—Gail Godwin

Educators are aware of the benefits of reviews and rehearsals to reinforce what is learned during class–that is, adult learners usually prefer active participation in the educational process (Bastable et al., 2010). Reviews and rehearsals may be used for each individual class, or for the entire childbirth class series (Carpenter et al., 2012). Whenever the class rejoins after a night or a week off, the educator should do a review to bring the class back to what was previously discussed. Likewise, prior to dismissal, there should be a wrap-up of the material learned during class. Of course, the most important review is one covering all the material learned throughout the class series (Nichols & Humenick, 2000). Below are some ideas for reviews and rehearsals to use with a childbirth class.

Mock Labor Scenarios

This review and rehearsal is one of the best ways to have the class members become aware of some events that may occur during labor and birth. It allows the class members to learn to master the information they have previously received. Role-playing may be the ideal teaching strategy for reviewing scenarios.

Create cards with various scenarios written on each one. Some scenarios should be quite basic to review the main concepts, such as determining when to go to the hospital, what stage or phase of labor the mother may be in, and demonstrating positions for use in certain phases of labor. Other scenarios should challenge their mastery of the material by giving specific problems and having them explain and demonstrate how they would respond. As an example, the couple must demonstrate how they would respond to being told the baby is in a posterior position and the caregiver is considering performing a cesarean delivery.

When creating the scenario cards, be sure to include both physical scenarios (ones involving the physical nature of labor and birth), as well as emotional issues surrounding labor and birth. The following are just a few examples of the endless possibilities for labor and birth scenarios.

- Contractions are 3 to 5 minutes apart, lasting 60 seconds, and you can no longer walk or talk through the contractions. You are at home, but plan to deliver at the hospital. What phase of labor are you likely in? Explain and/or demonstrate what you might do.

- Mother is having contractions that seemingly do not go away. She voices that she wants the contractions to end and she cannot take them anymore. What would you do?

- Mother was 8 cm when checked 15 minutes ago. During a contraction, she says she has to push, and begins to bear down and grunt. What would you do?

- Mother is working very hard during contractions and wants to have a natural childbirth. She is strong and determined, and vocalizes during contractions. Her mother, who wants to be at the birth, is telling her she is crazy for trying to go natural and she should get an epidural. How would you address this situation?

Term Cards to Review Labor Terms

There are numerous terms associated with labor and birth. In order for the couple to be fully informed about their options, they need to become familiar with these terms. As an exercise, you can place terms on index cards, and have the class members randomly pick cards and read the term to the rest of the class. Have the person/couple who picked the card explain what that term means, and its importance to pregnancy, labor, birth, or the postpartum period. Have the rest of the class give their input as well.

Some possible terms to include on the cards are: early labor, active labor, transition, AROM (artificial rupture of membranes), stripping the membranes, pitocin, prostaglandin, induction, electronic fetal monitoring, back labor, breech, pelvic station, effacement, dilation, lochia, colostrum, ring of fire, APGAR scoring, Bishop Score, perineum, and episiotomy.

Beach Ball Review

A fun way to review concepts learned during a class or series of classes involves an inflatable beach ball, which can be tossed around the room from class member to class member. To prepare for this exercise, purchase a standard, inflatable beach ball. With a permanent marker, write one activity on each colored panel.

You, as the teacher, verbally give a scenario to the class. Then toss the beach ball to one class member. Whoever catches the ball reads the activity on the section facing him/her and responds. If you are doing a review on labor and delivery, the actions on the ball may read:

- Choose one "labor tool" that may benefit.

- Demonstrate a position to use or suggest.

- Name one emotional need the mother might have at this time.

- State one way to change the environment.

- Identify a positive affirmation to say to the mother.

- Name one relaxation technique to try.

Once the person responds to the request or performs an action, he/she tosses the ball to someone else. Each person who catches the ball responds to the request facing him, even if someone else already responded to that request. There is more than one possible response for each. When you feel the particular scenario has been addressed adequately, you can go on to another scenario and continue the review. For suggestions on scenarios you may wish to use as the basis for this exercise, please refer to the Appendix.

Homework Assignment

No one likes homework, but all teachers know the value of learning outside of the classroom. You may find some of the class members will choose not to do the homework. The hope is that some will complete the work assignment. If giving a homework assignment, try to make it fun or interesting. Have them explore topics, such as medications and interventions. Perhaps give each couple a different intervention and ask them to present the intervention in class the next time they meet. If they know they will be called upon to contribute in class, then they likely will do the work outside of the classroom.

The Classic Game of Questions

The popular television gameshow where the answers are given in the form of questions is the format for this game. Use this to review a number of topics taught in a birthing or newborn class. For example, this topic will be Breastfeeding Basics.

Begin with a board or large surface where every-one can see. For each dollar box, there should be three layers of paper. Standard-sized pieces of paper work well for this. The top layer has the dollar amount, the middle layer has the question (answer), and the bottom layer would have answers for each question in the box. Remember, in this game, the answers are actually questions (See Diagram 5.1).

Let's Play Breastfeeding Basics

Nutrition	Anatomy & Positioning	Benefits	Pumping	Problems
$100	$100	$100	$100	$100
$200	$200	$200	$200	$200
$300	$300	$300	$300	$300
$400	$400	$400	$400	$400
$500	$500	$500	$500	$500

Diagram 5.1

To play, the class member would choose a category and a dollar amount. For example, the class member chooses Anatomy & Positioning for $100. You would tear off the first layer corresponding to the category and amount chosen, revealing the answer; "The part of the breast on which the baby latches." When a class member answers correctly, peal off that layer, exposing the question, "What is the areola?"

Once the board is completely revealed, the game is over. You may wish to offer a prize to the winner. This game may take a while to play, so be certain to allow enough time in your class curriculum.

Massage Demonstration with Feedback

Demonstrating massage is an integral part of any preparation for birth. The person usually responsible for massaging the laboring woman is her partner. Communication is essential for ensuring the type of massage the partner gives is one that feels good for the laboring woman. Practice time, prior to labor, is very important. Prior to pregnancy, a woman may simply enjoy the fact her partner is giving her a massage, but she doesn't verbalize how the massage could be more soothing for her if done in a different manner. For instance, some men have large, strong hands and can give a deep tissue massage. This may be good if that is what his partner prefers. However, if his partner is petite and prefers a more gentle massage, she may not be getting quite as much enjoyment out of it, even though she does not tell her partner this during class. Furthermore, during labor, she may actually verbalize the partner is hurting her and to stop touching her. If the partner and expectant mother communicate and practice massage before labor actually begins, they are better able to work in sync during the labor.

This exercise facilitates communication between the expectant mom and her partner with regards to massage. The mother is directed to give her partner a massage the way she would like a massage given to her. She should include verbal instructions to aid the partner in understanding her needs and desires. Upon completion of the massage, they switch roles. The partner now gives the massage the expectant mother explained and demonstrated to him.

The expectant mother is encouraged to communicate verbally and non-verbally to her partner so the partner can learn to master the technique. Discussions of room preparation and music preference should also coincide with the massage demonstration. After all, if the room is not comfortable for the expectant mother, and the music is not what she prefers, no matter how good the massage is, it will not be as effective.

Ice Contractions

When all of the techniques for relaxation, breathing, and comfort tools have been covered in class, practicing with "contractions" is one of the most effective ways to review and establish competency in the techniques.

Place several ice cubes in a plastic snap-lock sandwich bag. Prepare as many sandwich bags as there are expectant mothers in the class. Give a sandwich bag or "contraction" to the partner.

Explain that there will be two practice contractions using the "contraction." The first contraction will be for 45 seconds. Beginning with your verbal cue ("Contraction begins"), the partner places the "contraction" in the expectant mother's hand. During this 45 second contraction, the partner or mother should use effleurage or massage, rhythmical breathing, and focusing. Turn down the classroom lights, play pleasant, relaxing music, and perhaps provide some aromatherapy. When the contraction is over, again verbally cue the class ("Contraction ends"), and the ice is removed by the partner. Another 45 second contraction should be done. However, during the second contraction, no pain relief methods should be employed (for example: no specific breathing technique, no focusing, no massage, etc.). The ice should be placed in the expectant mother's other hand. At the end of this exercise, a noticeable difference will be noted by the expectant mother; the second contraction will seem longer and more uncomfortable.

You can choose to do the hard, unassisted contraction first followed by the one utilizing comfort measures to show what the comfort measures can actually do to minimize the intensity of the pain. Either way is effective for the review of techniques and provides a clear understanding of the Gate Control Theory.

Clothespins

One of the most challenging questions a birth educator hears is, "What do contractions feel like?" Expectant mothers often want to know about pain, and like having "practice contractions" while learning the various comfort measures they can use to handle the pain of labor. Ice contractions are one way to induce pain for practice purposes. Additionally, clothespins not only provide pain stimulation, but also help to explain what a contraction really is.

The expectant mother holds the clothespin in one hand using her thumb, index, and middle fingers. She begins by squeezing the clothespin and releasing it, quickly and repeatedly. After a short time, she will feel the contractions her arm muscles are making intensify. The longer she squeezes and releases the clothespin, the more pain she will eventually feel. Her muscles, in other words, cramp. Once she feels the burn of the muscles, have her release the clothespin. She will notice the pain from the contraction does not stop immediately, but actually decreases gradually.

This exercise is very similar to actual contractions. The uterus is made up of muscles. As they contract, the pain begins to intensify. After its peak, the contraction relaxes and the pain begins to wear off, like a wave. The clothespin demonstration emphasizes the "healthy and purposeful" pain of labor.

Michele Deck, BSN, MEd, LCCE, FACCE, has created a "cheer" to help parents remember certain comfort measures. She repeats this cheer frequently during her classes so that it is forever in their memories. The cheer, "PURE PEPSI," represents the physical and emotional comfort measures during labor.

Michele says, "Here is an example of a cheer I've used in childbirth education classes, but feel free to create your own that matches your content. I tell everyone when I say, "Hey, Hey" they must respond "PURE PEPSI." At intervals, when I see learners disinterested or nodding off, I say, "Hey, Hey." I repeat this technique until someone became curious enough to ask why were they saying, "PURE PEPSI."

Physical Comfort Measures

Position change (9 times out of 10, that makes some-one feel better.)

Urination (suggest she empty her bladder. When in labor, contractions mask the usual feel of urgency, and a full bladder can get in the way of a baby moving down and out.)

Relaxation (try one of the 6 ways to get her to re-lax, as stress hormone interfere with the body's flow of oxytocin, the hormone that gives a woman contrac-tions.)

Environment (you control her environment: if hot, fan her; if cold, cover her; turn light off/on as needed; no smelly food or coffee in room; regulate who is in room, according to her wishes.)

Emotional Comfort Measures

Praise (tell her every reason you care about her.)

Encourage (she needs to see and hear your confi-dence in her ability to birth.)

Perspective (a woman in labor has no time perspec-tive, don't try to predict or listen to predictions of how long this will take. Talk about what has happened al-ready; 9 hours of labor done.)

Support (support her efforts and decisions in labor, for you are her advocate.)

Inspiration (is there something of personal inspiration she wants and it is in her bag, such as a Bible, a rosary, or affirmations? Get it out and give it to her.)

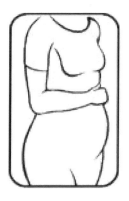

Chapter 7
Informed Consent and Interventions

Good teachers never teach anything. What they do is create the conditions under which learning takes place.

—S.I. Hayakawa

The subjects of medications and interventions can be some of the most difficult subjects to discuss with expectant parents. Every day, they are inundated with stories of bad birth experiences and outcomes from friends, family, and even total strangers. Television programs seem to indicate the use of medications and interventions are what birth usually involves. Expectant women hear over and over again how they are "crazy" to attempt to give birth to their baby without an epidural. Then, they read information from child-birth books and begin to learn more about options in birth. Now, they are more confused than ever. When teaching this subject, the educator has the responsibility to present accurate, non-biased information without leading them to fear the medication or procedure, should it become necessary.

Sometimes the best way to teach these subjects is to encourage the expectant parents to take an active role in the learning process. By researching and presenting their own information, they learn how to become informed consumers. The use of non-threatening teaching models aids in the learning process. By interjecting fun activities, such as games, grab bags, group work, and make-at-home teaching models, you can watch your class begin to own the material. Manipulatives help make abstract ideas concrete, since a picture says a thousand words.

Firsthand experience by handling items and viewing equipment close up can reduce the anxiety associated with heavy topics such as interventions. Remember from Chapter 1; maximum knowledge retention increases by combining various teaching strategies. Clients need a great understanding of interventions, and their risks and benefits. Therefore, it is especially wise to introduce games and models to drive home the information. In this section, you will find several ideas for teaching about medications and interventions with your clients.

Informed Consent

One way to teach with minimal bias is to teach using informed consent (ACOG, 2009; Goldberg, 2009).
Informed consent is a legal doctrine in America that is
defined in all 50 states as consent to treatment (for example, consent to a cesarean section or abdominal surgery to assist in the delivery of the baby) obtained after
adequate disclosure. As defined by Ethics in Medicine
from the University of Washington School of Medicine,
informed consent,

Five Questions of Informed Consent

1. What are the benefits to me, to my baby and
   to labor?

2. What are the risks to me, to my baby and to
   labor?

3. What are my alternatives?

4. What would happen if I did nothing?

5. Give me a moment to decide?

Diagram 7.1

Is the process by which a fully informed patient
can participate in choices about her health care. It orig-
inates from the legal and ethical right the patient has
to direct what happens to her body and from the ethical duty of the physician to involve the patient in her

health care (www.eduserv.hscer.washington.edu/bio-ethics/topics/consent.html.).

Before agreeing to any proposed treatment, the mother should be sure that the five questions of informed consent have been fully explained by her caregiver (See Diagram 6.1). Informed consent is not only beneficial for use in teaching about medications and interventions, but it can also be a life skill.

As mentioned in Chapter 4, educators also use acronyms for the five questions of informed consent, enabling parents to recall more efficiently. Acronyms, such as BRAN (Benefits, Risks, Alternatives, Now decide), BRAND (Benefits, Risks, Alternatives, Nothing, Decide), or BRAIN (Benefits, Risks, Alternatives, Intuition, Need time) can be used to present the information (Hodges, 2009; ICEA Informed Consent Discussion Sheet, 2008).

Medications Timeline

Fostering communication between the expectant mother and her partner is a vital role for the educator. Occasionally, they have differing opinions about the use of medication during labor and birth. To assist them in seeing any differences in opinion, and also to facilitate communication, print numerals 1 to 10 in a large font on 8.5 x 11 sheets of paper (brightly colored paper is fun). Tell class participants that "1" stands for "absolutely no medication," and "10" stands for having the "epidural mobile" visit the house before contractions begin.

Have the partners leave the room, and have the mothers stand by the number (and write down their choice on a piece of paper) best describing their feelings about medications during labor and birth. Then, have the mothers sit down and invite the partners back in to do the same; stand by the number that best describes their feelings about medications during labor and birth. Educators can vary this game by having the partners stand by the number they feel best describes their expectant mother's feelings.

What Will Your Partner Say?

This game is a test to show how well the partner and the expectant mother know each other. The partners and expectant mothers separate so that they cannot hear what the other one answers. Give the expectant mothers each a stack of tag board cards, cut to approximately 8.5 by 11 inches, and a marker with which to write. The number in each stack will depend on the number of questions you choose to ask.

You ask the expectant mothers a question and the moms need to answer how they think their partner will respond to that same question. A sample question may be, "What do you think your partner will say is the best way he/she can help you during labor?" The expectant mother then takes the marker and writes her answer on one card. Continue with the questions until all the questions have been answered.

Then invite the partners to join the mothers. Ask the partners questions, such as, "What is the best way you can help your wife/partner in labor?" Going one at a time, the partner responds to the question, and then the mother reveals what she previously wrote on the card. This is a fun game that emphasizes the importance of communication.

Name That Intervention

Prepare blank index cards with the printed definition of selected interventions. The definition might include the uses for the intervention, such as "to turn a persistent posterior baby" or "resembles salad tongs" for forceps, and can be as detailed as you wish. Hand one card per person, and invite each person to read their card and guess which intervention the definition describes. This game can be played with individuals, couples or teams, such as mothers vs. partners, or simply by dividing the class in half. To add to the longevity of the cards, you may wish to laminate the cards or use clear Contact™ paper for protection.

Create a List

In order to determine what expectant parents know about a particular subject, you can put a term, such as "epidurals," on the board, and ask them to each write a list of benefits and drawbacks on a piece of paper. When they have it completed, they can share their lists with their partners, and ultimately, the group, for further group discussions. You can assess what myths you may need to dispel, and provide explanations and clarifications on some of the information given from the participants.

Grab Bag of Interventions and More

Assemble a variety of interventions, including an amni-hook, epidural catheter, IV bag or line, external electronic fetal monitor transducers, internal electronic fetal monitor scalp electrode, intrauterine pressure catheter, Foley catheter, vacuum extractor, postpartum maxi pad, umbilical cord clamp, etc. Place these items in a decorative bag. Have participants "grab" an item without looking in the bag. Once all participants have an item, participants can tell the class about their item. If they do not know what their item is, they can ask for help from other members. Reinforce the discussion with charts and handouts for additional knowledge retention.

This activity, depending on the amount of class conversation, may take a long time to complete. You should plan plenty of time in your curriculum and monitor the conversations as you go along (for items and charts, visit Cascade Health or Childbirth Graphics).

Cesarean Teaching Aid

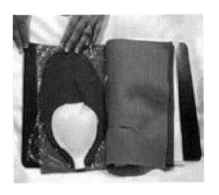

One of the challenges of teaching childbirth education classes is teaching about cesarean births. Videos can be expensive or too explicit. Charts also can be expensive, and words cannot accurately describe the actual procedure. It is, however, vital class that members understand that cesarean childbirth is a major abdominal surgery.

To aid in the explanation of cesarean birth, a felt teaching aid can be made. You will need:

Items Needed

- 10 pieces of felt (suggestions: one flesh color, white, two shades of red, green, yellow, two purple, a second flesh color, and blue)

- A piece of bubble wrap the size of the felt pieces

- A piece of plastic wrap cut to the size of the felt pieces

- A folder with two holes and a slider

- Scissors

- Hot glue gun

- ¾ Cup of oatmeal

- Small funnel

- Marker

- Pattern of fetus, uterus, and bladder (see Appendix)

Instructions for Assembly

With the marker, mark an umbilicus on the first flesh color piece of felt and make a Pfannenstiel incision (more commonly known in the United States as a "bikini cut," or low transverse incision) approximately eight inches from the umbilicus. Set this piece

aside. You may want to
add a layer of fat at this
point—this can be done
by adding a strip of bub-
ble wrap, the same size
as the other pieces of felt.

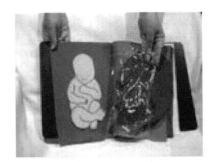

Make a "bikini cut"
on the white piece of felt,
as this represents the fascia. Set this piece aside. On the
two shades of red, make large cuts perpendicular to
the cut made on the fascia. These cuts represent the abdominal muscles that are separated during the surgical
procedure rather than cut. Set these pieces aside. Make
a "bikini cut" on the green piece of felt that represents
the peritoneum. Set this piece aside. Fold the yellow
piece of felt in half and place the bladder pattern on the
fold line. Cut out the bladder so the top of the bladder
is "hinged." Glue all sides together, leaving an open
space. Place the funnel inside of the open space and fill
the bladder with oatmeal. Glue the opening shut. Set
this piece aside. Trace the uterus onto the two purple
felt pieces and make a "bikini cut" on one. Trim plastic wrap to the same size as the rectangular felt pieces.
Trace the baby onto the second flesh color piece of felt.

Stack the felt pieces/shapes in the following order
from bottom to top: blue (rear of peritoneum), solid
piece of purple uterine-shaped felt, baby, plastic wrap,
piece of purple uterine shaped felt with "bikini cut,"
yellow bladder, green felt or peritoneum, both red

pieces, white felt, and finally, the flesh color felt. Make holes at the edge of the felt pieces so they can be inserted into the folder.

Episiotomy Tee

To illustrate how an episiotomy can actually cause perineal tearing, gather together an old tee-shirt and a pair of scissors. Show how during pushing, the perineum will stretch, and stretch a lot! Do this by using your two hands and pulling at opposite sides of the neck of the tee-shirt. Then mention that when an episiotomy is done (no matter how small), the simplest cut can greatly instigate a tear. Illustrate this by cutting along an imaginary line from the neck of the tee-shirt toward the body of the shirt. Demonstrate pushing after an episiotomy by again stretching the shirt. The shirt will tear along the line started by the cut.

Episiotomy with Polishing Cloth

Use a piece of polishing towelette; the type used in body shops and comes in 12 x 12 inch squares. Cut it into 16 equal squares. Fold each square into fourths. With each square, cut out a cone-shape (See Diagram 6.2), so when it opens, you have a hole in the middle of the square (See Diagram 6.3). In half of those, cut a small incision in the bottom of the circle. Half of the class gets one with a small cut and the others without. When demonstrating, use a baby doll and pretend its head is crowning and the towelette is the perineum. You may then show, with small scissors, how and where the cut is made, how the baby's head emerges, and causes the perineum to tear. Continue the demonstration by having the class try to stretch their circle as much as possible, showing how much easier it was for it to tear if there was already a cut.

Because this can be a graphic demonstration, use caution and assess your audience's ability to handle the visualization of cutting the perineum with scissors. You may need to do additional instruction, but it is important not to avoid the topic altogether. If an episiotomy is performed, they may see this in reality. Therefore, they may wish to be prepared for this in advance by doing this exercise.

What's on My Back?

Using large two-inch by two-inch Post-It Notes,™ write words such as "epidural," "forceps," "MityVac," and "amniotomy." Make as many Post-It Notes™ as there are class participants. When the time comes for this segment of the class, put a Post-It Note™ on the back of the participants without them seeing the note on their back. Others can look at the word and give the person hints as to what the term is on the Post-It Note™. It is up to the person to guess what the term is on their back by using questions which can be answered by "Yes" or "No." This teaching technique can also be used for postpartum or breastfeeding teaching.

The Domino Effect of Interventions

All birth educators should teach about the benefits, risks, and alternatives of various medical procedures. Undoubtedly, the risks include the need for other interventions. Therefore, it is important to explain the "Domino Effect of Interventions." The Domino Effect is one choice or procedure leading to the need for another, and so on. Other terms synonymous with this are "Cascade of Interventions," "Snowball Effect," or "Waterfall Effect"(Littleton-Gibbs & Engebretson, 2013; MacDonald, 2011; Goer & Romano, 2012).

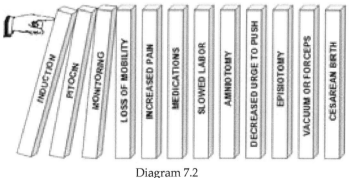

Diagram 7.2

Because this is an important topic for expectant parents to understand, as many interventions are directly linked to breastfeeding difficulties (Avery, 2013; Smith, 2009; Simkin et al., 2010), it is wise to not only explain the effect, but also to give a visual demonstration. To do this, use cereal boxes which have been covered with paper to cover up the box labels. Then, on the spine of each box, write an intervention. Line the boxes up in order like you would do with dominoes. Be sure that they are just far enough apart to cause them to fall down one by one when the first one is pushed over. The boxes can be labeled with the following interventions: Induction, Pitocin, Monitoring, Loss of Mobility, Increased Pain, Medications, Slowed Labor, Amniotomy, Decreased Urge to Push, Episiotomy, Vacuum or Forceps, and Cesarean Birth.

Waterfall Effect with Equipment

Ask for a volunteer from the class. You may wish to have the volunteer be a partner so he can feel what it may be like for the expectant mother to be constrained during labor. Have the volunteer sit in a chair, which simulates being bed-bound. Then one-by-one, add the equipment the laboring woman would most likely encounter when interventions are introduced into the labor process. While adding each piece, you can explain what they do, and why they may need to be introduced. Use equipment, such as the maternal and fetal monitors, blood pressure cuff, IV, oxygen mask, and an IV catheter with narcotics. Then talk about epidurals by taping the catheter to the volunteer's back, and then pretend to add Pitocin to the IV line for the decrease in contractions as a result of the epidural. You can then add the Foley catheter for urine output by taping it on the volunteer's leg (although, not everyone with an epidural gets one).

You do not need to use the actual equipment if they are not available. You can use yarn, string, or plastic tubing attached to the volunteer in the areas where they would actually be attached if the women were in the hospital. This is a very visual exercise that allows women and their partners to see how dependent they are during their labor, plus how incapable they are of moving around or actively participating in decision making.

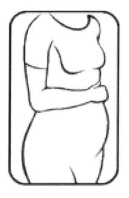

Chapter 8
Postpartum, Breastfeeding, and Infant Care

I tell women: Your body is not a lemon!

—Ina May Gaskin

Most new parents believe they will learn about their newborn from the Internet or in books. Little do they realize that on-the-job training is truly the best teacher. However, when teaching expectant parents about impending responsibilities with their newborns, it is not only important to make learning fun and memorable, but also to instill in them the fact that they do have resources to call upon after their precious bundle comes home.

Education about the postpartum period should also cover feeding methods. Continued research proves breast milk is the best food for babies of all ages. The American Academy of Pediatrics recommends exclusive breast milk for the first six months of a baby's life, and breastmilk and complementary foods after that (American Academy of Pediatrics, 2012). Breast milk is safer because it doesn't have to be mixed and is less likely to be contaminated. The baby does not have to wait for food as it is always the right temperature, and is an age-specific mixture that is always available at the mother's breast. Studies suggest babies who have been breastfed may be more intelligent and have fewer illnesses as they grow up (Huggins, 2015; Wiessinger et al., 2010).

Maternal benefits of breastfeeding include more rapid uterine involution, which is the return of the uterus to its pre-pregnant shape, and is influenced by the hormone oxytocin, which is stimulated by breastfeeding. Also, a closer relationship to the baby is experienced, as well as a feeling of satisfaction in being the sole source of food for the baby. Convenience and lack of expense are additional benefits (Newman & Pittman, 2006).

For a variety of reasons, which may or may not be disclosed to you, a mother may not wish to breastfeed her baby. Your role is to be supportive in the feeding decision. Make sure that the mother is confident in making and storing the formula, cleaning the bottles and nipples, and has access to clean water. If English is not the primary language of the mother, mixing directions should be made available in the client's native language. To enhance the experience, encourage the mother to hold the baby similar to a breastfeeding mother, and talk to and look at her baby. This emotional component is just as important as the nutritional component.

Helping a mother start off on the very best footing is one goal of an educator. Helping her achieve confidence in her mothering/parenting skills through supporting her decisions surrounding feeding her baby is important. Presenting a non-judgmental attitude, and being a consistent source of solid information can be the best support she'll receive.

Breastfeeding Basics

After the birth of the baby, estrogen and progesterone decrease, and levels of prolactin increase. Prolactin release is essential to milk production (Sears et al., 2013). The first nutrition the baby receives is called colostrum. It is higher in protein and lower in fat and lactose than mature milk. It also contains antibodies that protect the baby from illnesses as well as a laxative ingredient to help rid the baby's body of meconium. When the baby suckles at the breast, oxytocin is released by the posterior pituitary and the letdown

reflex occurs. Milk is propelled from the lactiferous sinuses to the nipple and into the baby's mouth.

A postpartum diet high in nutritious calories (approximately 300 to 500 calories more than her
normal diet), fluids (ap-proximately 64 fl oz), and
rest will enable the mother to breastfeed successfully
(Pryor & Huggins, 2007).

> *Weighing the baby before and after a feeding will give the number of ounces of breastmilk received at a feeding.*

However, if a mother is told she does not have enough
milk, or simply fears this, the let-down reflex may be
inhibited. If she gives her infant formula, there would
be less sucking stimulation and, consequently, a true
decrease in milk production. The best way to tell if
she has enough milk for the baby is to have her keep
a diaper diary, showing how many soiled diapers the
baby has each day.

Although the above information may not be enough
to convince some breastfeeding skeptics, a more accurate way of finding out how many ounces the baby is
receiving at a feeding is to weigh the baby before and
after a feeding. Prior to weighing, change the baby's
diaper. Weigh the baby on a professionally calibrated
scale and record the weight. Feed the baby normally,
using both breasts, allowing the baby to soil the diaper at will. Without changing the diaper, weigh the

baby. Subtract from this amount the weight prior to the feeding. This should give an ounces difference in weight and can be translated into the number of ounces of breast milk the baby has received at this feeding.

Many mothers prefer to sit or lie down to breastfeed their babies. No matter which position they choose, it should be a restful and relaxing time, with a glass of water available. The mother should be able to hold the baby without strain, and concentrate on this very precious gift she is giving her baby. The infant should be at the level of the breast, and not pull down on it or have to strain to reach the breast. One of the best suggestions for positioning is "baby to breast and chest to chest." This means the baby and the breast are on the same level, and both the baby's chest and the mother's chest are together. The baby should be able to grasp the nipple and the nipple is far back in the baby's mouth. If only the nipple is used to breastfeed, inadequate milk flow may occur, as well as creating sore nipples. Utilizing the rooting reflex to help the baby turn his/her head toward the mother and open the mouth can help get the baby on the breast properly.

Encourage the mother to talk to a lactation consultant during her stay at the birthing facility. The information that she will gain from speaking to the consultant will add to her self-esteem, educational base, and confidence in feeding her baby. Many lactation consultants will see new mothers after birth; they may practice in a clinic within a facility or in private practice in the community. Reinforce to the mother her choice was the very best choice for her and her baby. You may find that you are a significant support person for this new mother-baby dyad.

Diaper the Teddy Bear

Nothing is more fun in a parenting class than having each participant bring a teddy bear and learn positions for holding, swaddling, and diapering while using these non-threatening and cooperative little toys.

Have class participants bring their own teddy bear and a receiving blanket to class. Have available a package of disposable diapers at a local store, or even ask if the store could donate a package for parent education. Educators can instruct parents about the difference in cleaning the bottoms of little girls vs. little boys, how tightly to secure the diaper, and how to hold a baby. Mothers may also practice the different positions to breastfeeding with their bear.

If the timing is right, a discussion might begin on Shaken Baby Syndrome and Back Sleeping. Information about Shaken Baby Syndrome and Back Sleeping are included in the Resources Section of this book.

Grab Bag of Postpartum Care

Similar to the Grab Bag of Interventions found in Chapter 6, in a pillow case, assemble such items as a peri-bottle, postpartum hospital lochia pads, nursing bra, breast shields, infant nasal aspirator, hospital nametags, umbilical cord clamp, hospital bassinette name card, or term cards if the above items are not available. Pass around the pillow case and have each person take an item and share as much information as possible. Encourage other class members to share what they know about these items as well.

Normal Newborn Appearance

First-time parents benefit from not only hearing about certain newborn characteristics, but also from seeing them. Charts and slides available from birth education stores (Childbirth Graphics) are helpful in showing newborn appearance, characteristics, and procedures. However, you can inexpensively make charts and handouts by simply taking photographs yourself. If photographing a newborn, be sure to have consent, which includes the parents' signatures and permission to use their child's photo(s) for educational purposes. Take a series of pictures that capture as many newborn appearances as possible. Some suggestions for photos are: milia, cyanotic hands and feet swelling, rashes, stork bites/birth marks, and molding of the head.

Perhaps take pictures of newborn reflexes, as well as procedures. You may need to get permission from the hospital to take some pictures during procedures.

Over time, you can eventually gather a wide variety of pictures. Videos are also available to introduce parents to newborn appearances and characteristics. While some newborn procedures may vary from location to location, generally, videos can provide a safe learning experience.

Anatomically correct newborn models can be purchased and used for baby bath demonstrations, holding and bonding, and even practicing babywearing.

20 Questions

Often, expectant parents hesitate to ask questions during class because of the fear of looking uninformed or ignorant. To help get their questions answered anonymously, you can play the simple game of 20 Questions. Begin by handing out three blank index cards early during a class series. Have the couples write down one question per side of the card. No names should be put on the cards. During the final class, read the questions and answer them. This works well during an "end of class buffet party" time, and often facilitates other questions being asked.

Family Mobile

Many couples are uncertain of what life with a new baby will be like. You can demonstrate what to expect by bringing in a crib mobile. This works best with a mobile with objects arranged in a circle with four detachable pieces on the ends and one in the center.

At first, have only two pieces attached that are opposite one another. Tell the class,

> This represents you now, a mother and partner, whose life is relatively smooth and in balance. You have an established way of life that is basically in equilibrium. Then your baby comes along (attach a third piece to the mobile's circle, and the mobile becomes lopsided), and suddenly everything is thrown off! Life becomes out of balance, and temporarily will seem "off" for a while. This is normal, but is also temporary. The picture will be forever changed. In time, as you adjust to bringing the baby into the family, you will find a new normal and balance will be restored (move the third piece into the center, and the mobile is no longer lopsided). You, too, will find your "new normal" after the birth of your baby.

With the mobile, you can add another piece, and show what happens when you add an additional child. Once again, the balance will be temporarily thrown off.

When the newest baby is brought home and the family is complete (add that piece to the center), balance will be restored. This demonstration is a nice way to show expectant and new parents how they should expect some imbalance at first, but soon, the family will stabilize.

The Airplane Analogy

When discussing the postpartum period, you can teach parents how vital it is to take care of their health and nutrition. Give them a familiar analogy. Whenever we travel on an airplane, flight attendants give us the standard speech, "In the event of a drop in cabin pressure, you are to take the oxygen mask and place it on yourself first, before assisting your child."

Tell class members that there is a sound reason for this. If the parent does not first attend to their own vital needs, they will not be able to take care of their children's needs. The same is true of the postpartum period, when it is crucial to put a priority on getting enough food, drink, and rest, and to attend promptly to any physical or emotional difficulties. By doing this, parents ensure they will continue to be there to care for their baby's needs.

Make Your Own Breastfeeding Pillow

To make your own breastfeeding pillow for use in teaching about breastfeeding support, simply begin with a pair of small sweatpants. Sew the waist of the pants closed. Use pillow stuffing, or even plastic grocery bags, to stuff the sweatpants, leaving the bottom of the legs empty. This will enable the stuffed sweatpants to be wrapped around the waist and tie it closed. The stuffed body of the pillow should be in front. If teaching a large group, this is an inexpensive way to provide practice pillows for the class members.

Make a Breast Model

Educators often struggle with teaching about proper latch-on for breastfeeding. Posters can give a one-dimensional vision. However, having a model gives a better visualization of latch-on. Take a sheer, nylon knee-high stocking with a reinforced-toe foot and turn it inside out. Put enough knots on the seam and center of the reinforced toe so that when the sock is turned right-side-out, it looks like a nipple. Using brown or black thread, stitch around the lower outside of the nipple to allow it to stand out. If a model is needed to show inverted nipples, omit this stitching step.

Fill the remainder of the knee-high stocking with soft fiber batting until it is the shape of a breast. Since knee-high stockings come in a variety of shades, it is easy to make several breasts so cultural sensitivity can be included in the teaching of latch-on.

The Suck/Swallow Demonstration

All infants need to know how to suck, swallow, and breathe all at the same time in order for them to transfer milk from their mom and thrive. They can't successfully transfer the milk if they are positioned and latched incorrectly. Improper latch-on causes one of the most common breastfeeding complaints; sore nipples, which can lead to a host of breastfeeding problems or early weaning if not corrected quickly.

Sometimes adults cannot quite grasp the idea of proper latch-on unless they actually experience it. Here is a trick that mothers can do to concretely understand how babies need to be positioned and latched to eat.

Purchase the following supplies for each class member.

Supplies Needed Per Participant

- 1 small cup of water (or water bottle) that can have a straw inserted into it

- 1 straw

Procedure

1. Ask your mothers to insert their straws into their cups. If you are providing them with a water bottle with a pull-up cap, no straw will be needed.

2. Tell them to turn their heads all the way to one side, looking at their shoulder.

3. Have them try to take a drink from their straws or bottles with their heads turned to the side. There may be hard gulping noises, or comments that they cannot do it at all.

4. Ask them to remember how they were sucking and how their tongues worked to wrap around the straw or bottle.

5. Now ask them to face forward and take a drink of their water. They should be able to do this easily.

6. Ask them if they noticed a difference and what it was.

7. Tell them that their first experience in drinking turned sideways is an example of bad positioning, because it's harder to drink when not turned in the direction of the natural position of the body.

8. Ask them if they liked it better when drinking facing forward. This is how the baby likes it, too.

9. Let them know that babies whose heads are not in alignment with their abdomen and buttocks cannot eat properly.

Ask them to remember how they sucked when their heads were turned sideways. It is harder to transfer liquids this way, and they may not have been properly latched onto the straw. Their tongues may not have gotten farther back on the straw with their heads turned.

Another way to use this technique is to teach asymmetrical latch. This can be taught by omitting the straw from their drinks.

1. Ask them to drink in a straight line with their cups. This can be achieved by having their heads look directly in front of them with no tilt to their heads.

2. Next, ask them to tilt their heads slightly backwards, as if naturally drinking from a cup of

water, as they tilt their heads back to get more liquid into their bodies.

3. Ask them which technique allowed them to drink their water faster and in higher quantity.

4. Did they feel they got more from tilting their heads back? Did their chin touch the cup?

5. This is how babies' heads need to be: slightly tilted back about 10 degrees with their chins touching the underside of breast, lips flanged surrounding more of the lower areola (an off-center latch or asymmetrical latch), to get more milk transferred into their stomachs.

Some educators may feel more comfortable using cups of water instead of bottled water to de-emphasize bottles. The less the word "bottle" in the context of learning how to breastfeed is used, the better. Of course, if cups are not available and they have their own drinks or bottled water, they can use that to learn.

Perinatal Mood and Anxiety Disorders

With between 15% to 25% of new mothers experiencing postpartum mood and anxiety disorders (PMAD) in the first year following childbirth, it is important to cover this topic with parents. The debilitating effects of PMAD on the new mother's life and the new family may seem far and distant from those who sit in a childbirth education class (Bennett & Indman, 2015; Honikman, 2014).

Education may help in reducing the stigma associated with PMAD. This is as important for the partner as it is for the new mother because it is often the partner who first sees the signs or symptoms. Encourage parents to include a Postpartum Circle of Healing (Morelli, 2013) in their birth plan in an effort to identify sources of support during the postpartum time, especially if there are extreme circumstances. With this, plan for infant feeding, guest visitation, social support, community resources, and professional support, and be written and clear.

During discussion about the postpartum time and PMAD, the role of the Postpartum Doula can also be introduced. While self-efficacy is encouraged for the laboring/birthing mother, few conversations bring up what happens after the birth. The feelings of being overwhelmed and insufficient begin to overcome any previous feelings of empowerment and suddenly, the new mother is lost in a sea of tears and emotions. Postpartum doula care has a positive impact on breast-feeding rates, parent-infant bonding, emotional recovery, and helping women find their instinctual talents as mothers (Pascali-Bonaro et al., 2014).

Adjusting to life with a new baby, older children and a partner have unique challenges. Things will not "get back to normal," but rather, there will be a "new normal" for parents to discover (Taylor, 2014). Providing a list of Internet resources and books will help parents to have sources to look back on and get help.

Guest Speaker(s) or Panel Discussions

Parents often learn best from their peers. Invite new parents and their babies from previous classes to come to a "sharing time" during class. The veteran parents can share helpful hints, their experiences, and let the still pregnant couples know first-hand how the information is beneficial and usable.

Regardless of whether the classes are taught privately or for a birthing facility, the educator may invite a pediatrician for a question-and-answer session. Be aware, however, that whomever is chosen for whatever topic, may appear to indicate favoritism.

Lactation professionals and La Leche League leaders also make good guest speakers. Note that these two groups of individuals are obviously pro-breastfeeding. Therefore, those in class who choose not to breastfeed may not want to attend. It is best to make this class or section of class optional, but include handouts with the regular set of handouts or manual.

For covering difficult topics, such as PMAD, guest speakers who are community experts can take the pressure off of the educator and link parents to resources which they may have been unaware of.

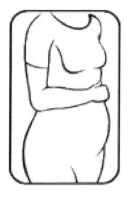

Chapter 9
Closings

It is good to have an end to journey toward;
but it is the journey that matters, in the end.

—Ursula K. LeGuin

When childbirth classes end, sometimes parents have difficulty. They have bonded with the educator, and recognized how much they didn't know. Parents enjoy the time with peers, especially when they have made friends in the class. Bringing a class to a close may also be difficult with the educator when she/he has also bonded with the class members.

Guest Speaker Panel

As mentioned previously, having guest speakers or a speaker's panel discussion not only takes the pressure off of the educator, but also allows the class members to hear the same information from another reputable source. This validates the educator and the information presented. Plus, seeing new parents and their babies make childbirth "real" for those in the class.

Be sure that the guest(s) understand time limitations and any ground rules before they arrive. Present specific instructions on what time to arrive, the parking situation, and the actual location of the class. Arrange with the speaker what will happen if a question is asked that they would rather not answer. The educator can take control of the situation and diffuse the pressure on the guest.

Potluck

Nothing brings people together quite like food. An end-of-class potluck should be anything but potluck. Planning a variety of foods (avoiding repeats) and eliminating the possibility of food allergies is essential. The first night of class, announce that there will be a potluck at the last class. Prompt members to sign up for healthy food items plus paper plates, cups, and napkins, if necessary.

172

Candle-Lighting Ceremony

At the end of the class or workshop, have a table ready with a large pillar candle on a charger plate, fireplace matches or butane lighter with flexible neck, a taper candle, and as many tea light candles as there are class/workshop participants. You can find small holders in a variety of colors for tea lights at stores where candles are sold. Have the participants stand around the table with the pillar candle/charger in the middle. A round table works well. Have a tea light and one fireplace match in front of each participant. Light the taper candle and express your feelings about the class/workshop. Pass the taper candle to a participant and invite them to share their feelings, and then light their tea light from the taper candle. This continues until the all participants have lit their tea lights. Then tell the participants to pick up the fireplace match and from their tea light flames, light the larger pillar candle. This signifies that they were once individuals, but are now part of a larger cohesive group.

Dream Catcher

This is ideal for a large group of highly motivated individuals, such as fellow colleagues at a workshop. It can also work for a childbirth education class, especially if they have all bonded closely. Assemble three to five colors of yarn in balls. Arrange the group in a large circle. Select three to five individuals as the starting points and tell them to begin tossing the balls back and forth within the group, crisscrossing. Each individual, including the first set of individuals, needs to keep a hold of their piece of yarn while throwing the yarn ball around the room. After a web, or Dream Catcher, has formed, tell the group that at the beginning, they all began as individuals from different back-grounds. Now they all share something special that connects them. Continue by adding unique observations from the class or workshop. Cut pieces of the dream catcher for all to take with them.

Class Photo/Social Media

A great keepsake from a childbirth education class are class photos. If using the photos for promotional use or on social media, consider using a standard photo release form, granting permission from those in the photo for their image to be used.

Social media is also a great way to stay connected with class members. However, a public page on Facebook might be too public for some. Consider a "closed" Facebook page for your classes so that members can keep in touch, ask questions, and feel connected. Maintaining the privacy of the new family is extremely important.

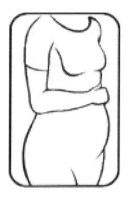

Appendix
Suggested Scenarios for Reviews and Rehearsals

For Doula Trainers

1. You have a client stalled at 5-6 cm.

2. Your client complains of pain in her lower back, especially during contractions.

3. Your client calls and says she is tired of being pregnant. She is 40+ weeks gestation and considering induction.

4. Your primip client is 32 weeks and has intermittent contractions.

5. At 39 weeks, after a complicated pregnancy, your client decides to have a cesarean delivery.

She says she no longer needs a doula, and asks for her money back.

6. Your client's mother is not supportive of your client's wishes, and is making negative side-comments. Prenatally, the client stated she wanted her mom to be there.

7. There are four patients in active labor and one nurse on duty because the other is at lunch. Your client has to push.

8. Your client responds well to vocalization, yet her doctor tells her to stop making noise during the pushing stage.

For Birthing Classes

1. Mother is having sporadic lower back pain and irregular contractions, and it is 10 p.m. What should you do? If the time was 9 a.m., would you do anything differently?

2. Mother is experiencing contractions at 4 to 6 minutes apart and lasting 1 minute. She is getting increasingly more uncomfortable and is at home. She plans to deliver at the hospital.

3. Mother's labor is slowing down, and her caregiver expresses concern. The caregiver wants to start Pitocin in an hour or so if labor does not

kick in. What can you do to try to get labor going again?

4. Mother has expressed that she does not want pain medications, and that you, her partner, need to support her decision, no matter what. You are not to waiver on this decision she made. During labor she begs for medication, and says to disregard what she said earlier. Now what do you do?

5. Mother is trembling, hiccupping, and experiencing hot and cold flashes. Her contractions are 2 to 3 minutes apart, and lasting 60 to 90 seconds. She is expressing, "I cannot do this" and "help me." What would you do?

6. Mother has intense lower back pain that does not go away between contractions. Demonstrate positions she can use to both correct the situation and minimize the pain.

7. Mother begins to grunt and states that she has to push. She has not been given a vaginal exam in a while. What do you do and what breathing would you suggest?

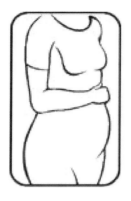

References

ACOG Committee Opinion No. 439. Informed Consent. (2009) American College of Obstetricians and Gynecologists. *Obstetrics Gynecology, 114,* 401–408.

American Academy of Pediatrics Policy Statement (2012). Breastfeeding and the use of human milk. *Pediatrics, 129*(3), e827 -e841.

Amis, D., & Green, J. (2014). *Prepared childbirth: The educator's guide.* Plano, TX: Family Way Publications.

Avery, M. (2013). *Supporting a physiologic approach to pregnancy and birth: A practical guide.* Hoboken, NJ: Wiley-Blackwell.

Baldwin, R. (1995). *Special delivery.* Berkeley, CA: Celestial Arts.

Bastable, S., Gramet, P., Jacobs, K., & Sopczyk, D.L. (2010). *Health professional as educator: Principles of teaching and learning.* Sudbury, MA: Jones & Bartlett Learning.

Bean, C. (1974). *Methods of childbirth: A complete guide to childbirth classes and maternity care.* Garden City, NY: Dolphin Books.

Beiranvand, S., Noparast, M., Eslamizade, N., & Saeedikia, S. (2014). The effects of religion and spirituality on postoperative pain, hemodynamic functioning and anxiety after cesarean section. *Acta Medica Iranica, 52*(12), 909-915.

Bennett, S., & Indman, P. (2015). *Beyond the blues: Understanding and treating prenatal and postpartum depression and anxiety.* San Francisco: Untreed Reads Publishing.

Benson, H., & Klipper, M. (2000). *The relaxation response.* New York: Harper Torch/Reissue Edition.

Bing, E. (1994). *Six practical lessons for an easier childbirth, 3rd Edition.* New York: Bantam Books.

Bradley, R. (2008). *Husband coached childbirth. 5th Edition.* New York: Bantam Books.

Brady, C. (2013) Understanding learning styles: Providing the optimal learning experience. *International Journal of Childbirth Education, 28*(2), 16-19.

Buckley, S. (2015), *Hormonal physiology of childbearing: Evidence and implications for women, babies and maternity care.* Washington, DC: Childbirth Connection. http://childbirthconnection.org/pdfs/CC.NPWF.HPoC.Report.2015.pdf

Carpenter, S.K., Cepeda, N.J., Rohrer, D., Kang, S.H.K., & Pashler, H. (2012). Using spacing to enhance diverse forms of learning: Review of recent research and implications for instruction. *Educational Psychology Review, 24*, 369-378.

Charles, A.G., Norr, K.L., Block, C.R., Meyering, S., & Meyers, E. (1978). Obstetric and psychological effects of psychoprophylactic preparation for childbirth. *American Journal of Obstetrics and Gynecology, 131*(1), 44-52.

Chlup, D., & Collins, T.E. (2010). Breaking the ice: Using icebreakers and re-energizers with adult learners. *Adult Learning, 21*(3), 34-39.

Clark, M.E., McCorkle, R.R., & Williams, S.B. (1981). Music therapy assisted labor and delivery. *Journal of Music Therapy, 28*(2), 88-100.

111111111

11111111111111111111111111111111111111

Declercq, E. R., Sakala, C., Corry, M.P., Applebaum, S. (2006). *Listening to Mothers II: Report of the second national U.S. survey of women's childbearing experiences.* Washington, DC: Childbirth Connection.

Dick-Read, G. (2013). *Childbirth without fear: The principles and practice of natural childbirth, 2nd Ed.* London: Pinter & Martin.

DiFranco, J.T., & Curl, M. (n.d.). *Avoid giving birth on your back, and follow your body's urges to push.* Retrieved from: http://www.lamazeinternational.org/p/cm/ld/fid=214

Doula Office 2.2. (2014) Perinatal Education Associates, Inc.

Edmonton Symptom Assessment Scale. Retrieved from: http://www.npcrc.org/files/news/edmonton_symptom_assenssment_scale.pdf.

Frey, H.A., Tuuli, M.G., Cortez, S., Odibo, A.O., Roehl, K.A., Shanks, A.L., Macones, G.A., & Cahill, A.G. (2012). Does delayed pushing in second stage of labor impact perinatal outcomes. *American Journal of Perinatology, 29*(10), 807-814. doi: 10.1055/s-0032-1316448.

Frey, H.A., Tuuli, M.G., Cortez, S., Odibo, A.O., Roehl,

K.A., Shanks, A.L., Macones, G.A., & Cahill, A.G. (2013). Medical and non-medical factors influencing utilization of delayed pushing in second stage. *American Journal of Perinatology, 30*(7), 595-600. doi: 10.1055/s-0032-1329689

Gizzo, S., Di Gangi, S., Noventa, M., Bacile, V., Zambon, A., & Nardelli, G.B. (2014). Women's choice of positions during labour: Return to the past or a modern way to give birth? A cohort study in Italy. *BioMed Research International,* 638093. doi:10.1155/2014/638093

Goer, H., & Romano, A. (2012). *Optimal care in childbirth: The case for a physiologic approach.* Seattle, WA: Classic Day Publishing.

Goldberg, H. (2009). Informed decision making in maternity care. *Journal of Perinatal Education, 18*(1), 32-40.

Grossman E., Grossman, A., Schein, M.H., Zimlichman, R., & Gavish, B. (2001). Breathing-control lowers blood pressure. *Journal of Human Hypertension, 15*(4), 263-269.

Hodges, S. (2009). Abuse in the hospital-based birth settings. *Journal of Perinatal Education, 18*(4), 8-11. doi: 10.1624/105812409X474663.

Honikman, J. (2014). *I'm listening: A guide to support-ing postpartum families.* Amazon Digital Services. Retrieved from: http://www.amazon.com/Im-Listening-Supporting-Postpartum-Families/dp/0692305807

Huggins, K. (2015). *The nursing mother's companion,7th Ed.: The breastfeeding book mothers trust, from preg-nancy through weaning.* Boston: Harvard Common Press.

ICEA. (2008). *ICEA informed consent discussion sheet.* Retrieved from: https://www.icea.org/sites/de-fault/files/informed%20consent.pdf

ICEA Position Paper. (2014). The role and scope of birth doula practice. (2014). Retrieved from: http://www.icea.org/sites/default/files/Role%20&%20Scope%20of%20Doula%20PP-FINAL.pdf

ICEA Position Paper. (2014). *Water labor, water birth.* Re-trieved from: http://www.icea.org/sites/default/files/Water%20Birth.pdf

Icebreaker list from Wayne State University. http://lc.wayne.edu/pdf/icebreakers_teambuilders.pdf

Karmel, M. (2005). *Thank you, Dr. Lamaze: A mother's ex-periences in painless childbirth- revised.* Garden City,

NY: Dolphin Books.

Kitzinger, S. (1979). *Education and counseling for childbirth.* New York: Schocken Books.

Kitzinger, S. (2003). *The complete book of pregnancy and childbirth.* New York: Knopf Publications.

Kitzinger, S. (2004). *The new experience of childbirth.* Sussex, UK: Orion Books.

Kitzinger, S. (2011). *The new pregnancy and childbirth; Choices and challenges.* London: Dorling Kindersley Limited.

Knowles, M., Holton, E., Swanson, R., & Holton, E. (1998). *The definitive classic in adult education and human resource development.* Houston, TX: Golf Publishing Company.

Kolb, D. (1984). *Experiential learning.* Englewood Cliffs, NJ: Prentice-Hall.

Kolb, D.A. (1985). *Learning style inventory.* Boston: McBear and Company.

Kwan, W.S.C., Chan, S-W., & Li, W-H. (2011). The Birth Ball experience: Outcome evaluation of the intrapartum use of birth ball. *Hong Kong Journal of Gynecology, Obstetrics, and Midwifery, 11*, 59-64.

Livingston, C. (2014). *The birth ball source book.* Dayton, OH: Birth-source.

Littleton-Gibbs, L., & Engebretson, J. (2013). *Maternity nursing, 2nd Ed.* San Francisco: Cengage Learning.

Liu, Y., Liu, Y., Huang, X., Du, C., Peng, J., Huang, P., & Zhang, J. (2014). A comparison of maternal and neonatal outcomes between water immersion during labor and conventional labor and delivery. *BMC Pregnancy and Childbirth, 14:160.* doi: 10.1186/1471-2393-14-160.

Lothia, J., & De Vries, C. (2010). *The official Lamaze guide: Giving birth with confidence, 2nd Ed.* Minnetonka, MN: Meadowbrook Press.

MacDonald, C. (2011). *The cascade of intervention: How one medical intervention can lead to many more.* Retrieved from: http://birthissues.org/education/508-2/

Maslow, A. (1943). A theory of human motivation. *Psychological Review, 50*, 370-396.

Melzack, R., & Wall, P. (1965). Pain mechanisms: *A new theory. Science, 150*(3699), 971-979.

Mendelson C. L. (1946) The aspiration of stomach contents into the lungs during obstetric anaesthesia. *American Journal of Obstetrics and Gynaecology, 52,* 191–205.

Morelli, K. (2013). *BirthTouch® pocket guide to perinatal mental illnesses for childbirth educators.* Retrieved from: http://www.amazon.com/BirthTouch%C2%AE-Perinatal-Illness-Childbirth-Educators-ebook/dp/B00BEUESG2

My Plate Nutritional Information for Pregnancy. Retrieved from: http://www.choosemyplate.gov/mypyramidmoms/

Namazi, M., Akbari, A.A., Mojab, F., Talebi, A., Alavi Majd, H., & Jannesari, S. (2014). Aromatherapy with citrus aurantium oil and anxiety during the first stage of labor. *Iran Red Crescent Medical Journal, 16*(6), e.18371. doi: 10.5812/ircmj.18371.

Newman, J., & Pitman, T. (2006). *The ultimate breastfeeding book of answers: The most comprehensive problem-solving guide to breastfeeding from the foremost expert in North America, revised and updated edition.* New York: Harmony Publishing.

Nichols, F., & Humenick, S. (2000). *Childbirth education: Practice, research, and theory. 2nd. Ed.* Philadelphia: W.B. Saunders.

Odent, M. (2000). Insights into pushing: Second stage as a disruption of the fetus ejection reflex. *Midwifery Today International Midwife, 55,* 12.

Pascali-Bonaro, D., Arnold, J., Ringel, M., & Lathrop, K. (2014). *Nurturing beginnings: Guide to postpartum care for doulas and community outreach workers.* Retrieved from: http://www.amazon.com/Nurturing-Beginnings-Postpartum-Community-Outreach-ebook/dp/B00JGVZJOQ

Pryor, G., & Huggins, K. (2007). *Nursing mother, working mother – Revised: The essential guide to breastfeeding your baby before and after your return to work.* Boston: Harvard Common Press.

Schwartz, L., Toohill, J., Creedy, D.K., Baird, D.K., Gamble, J., & Fenwick, J. (2015). Factors associated with childbirth self-efficacy in Australian childbearing women. *BMC Pregnancy and Childbirth, 15*:29. doi: 10.1186/s12884-015-0465-8.

Sears, W., Sears, M., Holt, L., & Snell, B.J. (2013). *The healthy pregnancy book: Month by month, everything you need to know from America's baby experts.* New York: Little, Brown and Co.

Sears, W., Sears, M., Sears, R., & Sears, J. (2013). *The baby book, Revised Ed. Everything you need to know about your baby from birth to age two.* New York: Little, Brown and Co.

Simkin, P., Whalley, J., Keppler, A., Durham, J., & Bolding, A. (2010) *Pregnancy, childbirth and the newborn: The complete guide.* Minnetonka, MN: Meadowbrook Press.

Simpson, K.R. (2006). When and how to push: Providing the most current information about second-stage labor to women during childbirth education. *Journal of Perinatal Education, 15*(4), 6-9.

Simavli, S., Kaygusuz, I, Gumus, I, Usluogullari, B., Yildirim, M., & Kafali, H. (2014). Effect of music therapy during vaginal delivery on postpartum pain relief and mental health. *Journal of Affective Disorders, 156*, 194-199. doi: 10.1016/j.jad.2013.12.027.

Sinqata, M., Tranmer, J., & Gyte, G.M.L. (2013). *Restricting oral fluid and food intake during labor.* Cochrane Database for Systematic Review. Retrieved from: DOI: 10.1002/14651858.CD003930.pub3

Smith, L.J., & Kroeger, M. (2009). *Impact of birthing practices on breastfeeding, 2nd Ed.* Sudbury, MA: Jones & Bartlett Learning.

Sprague, A. (2011). *Water labour water birth: a guide to the use of water during childbirth.* Retrieved from: http://www.amazon.com/WATER-LABOUR-BIRTH-childbirth-pregnancy-ebook/dp/B0052LFX6S

Stadtlander, L. (2013). How learning works: Application for childbirth education. *International Journal of Childbirth Education, 28*(2), 12-15.

Taavoni, S., Abdolahian, S., Haghani, H., & Neysani, L. (2011). Effect of birth ball usage on pain in the active phase of labor: A randomized controlled trial. *Journal of Midwifery and Women's Health, 56*(2), 137-140. doi: 10.1111/j.1542-2011.2010.00013.x.

Taylor, E. (2014). *Becoming us: 8 steps to grow a family that thrives.* Harper/Collins Australia/New Zealand: Three Turtles Press.

University of Washington School of Medicine: Ethics in medicine. Retrieved from: http://eduserv.hscer.washington.edu/bioethics/topics/consent.html.

Waller-Wise, R. (2013). Utilizing Henderson's Nursing Theory in childbirth education. *International Journal of Childbirth Edu-cation, 28*(2), 30-34.

Wiessinger, D., West, D., & Pitman, T. (2010). *The womanly art of breastfeeding – La Leche League International, 8th Ed.* London: Pinter and Martin LTD.

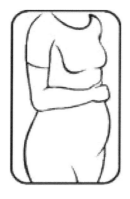

Online Resources

Academy of Breastfeeding Medicine
Worldwide organization of physicians dedicated
to the promotion, protection and support of
breastfeeding and human lactation.
www.bfmed.org
1 -914-740-2115

American Academy of Pediatrics
www.aap.org

American College of Nurse-Midwives
www.midwife.org

American Congress of Obstetricians and
Gynecologists
www.acog.org

Association of Women's Health Obstetrics and
Neonatal Nursing
Position Statements and more
www.awhonn.org

Australian College of Midwives
National, nonprofit serves as peak professional body
for midwives in Australia.
www.midwives.org.au

Bright Future Lactation Resource Centre Ltd.
Linda J. Smith
www.bflrc.com

Canadian Foundation for the Study of Infant Deaths
"Baby's Breath"
www.sidscanada.org

Cascade Health Care Products
Resource for pelvis and baby models; grab bag items
www.1cascade.com/
1-800-443-9942

Center for Disease Control (Folic Acid) http://www.
cdc.gov/ncbddd/folicacid/recommendations.html

Childbirth Connection (formerly Maternity Center
Association)
Evidence-based documents, handouts, pamphlets.
www.childbirthconnection.org

Childbirth Graphics
www.childbirthgraphics.com
1-855-510-6730

Childbirth and Parenting Educators of Australia
Not for profit professional organization supporting
birth and parenting educators in Australia.
www.capea.org.au

Coalition for Improving Maternity Services
Home of Mother-Friendly Childbirth Initiative
www.motherfriendly.org

DONA International
Birth & Postpartum Doula Certification
www.dona.org
1-888-788-DONA

Express Yourself Mums
Leading UK Supplier of Baby Products
www.expressyourselfmums.co.uk

Family Paws Parent Education
Offering families and professionals specialized
resources and support to increase safety and success
with family dog as baby grows.
http://www.familypaws.com
1-877-247-3407
jen@familypaws.com

International Board of Lactation Consultant
Examiners
www.iblce.org

International Cesarean Awareness Network
www.ican-online.org
1-800-686-ICAN

International Childbirth Education Association
(ICEA)
Evidence-based Position Papers, multiple
certifications (professional childbirth educator, birth
and postpartum doula) and certificate programs
(nutrition, perinatal exercise, lactation) all with
nursing CEs, Bookstore.
www.icea.org
1-919-863-9487

International Lactation Consultant Association
Worldwide network of lactation professionals
www.ilca.org

International MotherBaby Childbirth Organization
Nonprofit organization to update and promote
International MotherBaby Childbirth Initiative: 10
Steps to Optimal Maternity Services Worldwide.
www.imbci.org
1-904-285-0028

Lamaze International
Childbirth certification; Healthy Birth Practices
www.lamazeinternational.org
1-800-368-4404

La Leche League International
Breastfeeding information
www.llli.org
1-800-LALECHE

Massachusetts Breastfeeding Coalition
Excellent resource for breastfeeding materials
www.massbreastfeeding.org

Midwives Alliance of North America
Professional midwifery association promoting the
Midwifery Model of Care.
www.mana.org

Mothers' Advocate
Online joint venture between Injoy Birth and
Parenting and Lamaze International, providing free
videos and professionally designed handouts.
www.mothersadvocate.org

National Association of Certified Professional
Midwives
CPMs have met the standards for certification by the
North American Registry of Midwives (www.narm.
org)
www.nacpm.org

National Center on Shaken Baby Syndrome
www.dontshake.com

National Institute of Child Health & Human
Development, SIDS: "Back to Sleep" Campaign
www.nichd.nih.gov/sids

Optimal Care in Childbirth
Website for Amy Romano and Henci Goer's landmark
book: *Optimal Care in Childbirth: The Case for a
Physiologic Approach.*
www.optimalcareinchildbirth.com

Perinatal Education Associates, Inc.
Offers evidence-based information for parents and
professionals.
www.birthsource.com
Toll free 1-866-88-BIRTH (US only)
1-937-312-0544

Postpartum Progress
Links to worldwide organizations offering support
for perinatal mood and anxiety disorders.
www.postpartumprogress.com

Postpartum Support International
Excellent resource for Perinatal Mood and Anxiety
Disorders
www.postpartum.net
1-800-944-4773

Royal College of Obstetricians and Gynaecologists
www.rcog.org.uk
+44 20 7772 6200

Shaken Baby Alliance
www.shakenbaby.com

Stigmama
Research based website on perinatal mood and
anxiety disorders; website of author Dr. Walker
Karraa.
http://www.drwalkerkarraa.com/stigmama-1.html

Texas Tech University Health Sciences Center
Dr. Thomas Hale/Breastfeeding
www.infantrisk.com

Twin to Twin Transfusion Syndrome Foundation
www.tttsfoundation.org
1-800-815-9211

United States Breastfeeding Committee
Independent nonprofit coalition of more than 50
nationally influencial professional, education and
governmental organizations.
www.usbreastfeeding.org

VBAC.COM
Outstanding resource on Vaginal Birth After
Cesarean; website of researcher and author, Nicette
Jukelevics.
www.vbac.com

VBAC Facts
Website of Jen Kamel, VBAC expert and activist
www.vbacfacts.com

World Alliance for Breastfeeding Action
Global network of individuals and organizations
supporting the Innocenti Declaration and the
Global Strategy for Infant and Young Child Feeding.
Sponsor of World Breastfeeding Week.
www.waba.org.my
604-6584816

World Health Organization
Multiple worldwide fact sheets
www.who.int/topics/pregnancy/en

Zip Milk
Need breastfeeding support? Just enter zip code.
www.zipmilk.org

Printed in Great Britain
by Amazon.co.uk, Ltd.,
Marston Gate.